A Field Guide to the
Huángdì Nèijīng Sùwèn

of related interest

Grasping the Donkey's Tail
Unraveling Mysteries from the Classics of Oriental Medicine
Peter Eckman, MD, PhD, MAc (UK)
Foreword by Charles Buck, MSc, BSc, BAc
ISBN 978 1 84819 351 2
eISBN 978 0 85701 310 1

Foundations of Theory for Ancient Chinese Medicine
Shang Han Lun and Contemporary Medical Texts
Guohui Liu, MMed, LAc
Foreword by Charles Buck
ISBN 978 1 84819 262 1
eISBN 978 0 85701 211 1

Gold Mirrors and Tongue Reflections
The Cornerstone Classics of Chinese Medicine Tongue Diagnosis—
The Ao Shi Shang Han Jin Jing Lu, and the Shang Han She Jian
Ioannis Solos
Forewords by Professor Liang Rong and Professor Chen Jia-xu
ISBN 978 1 84819 095 5
eISBN 978 0 85701 076 6

A Field Guide to the

Huángdì Nèijīng
黃帝內經素問 **Sùwèn**

A Clinical Introduction to the Yellow Emperor's
Internal Classic, Plain Questions

Amy Chang

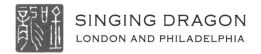

SINGING DRAGON
LONDON AND PHILADELPHIA

First published in Great Britain in 2021 by Singing Dragon,
an imprint of Jessica Kingsley Publishers
An Hachette Company

1

Copyright © Amy Chang 2021

The right of Amy Cheng to be identified as the Author of the Work has been
asserted by her in accordance with the Copyright, Designs and Patents Act 1988.

The information contained in this book is not intended to replace the services of trained medical
professionals or to be a substitute for medical advice. The complementary therapy described in
this book may not be suitable for everyone to follow. You are advised to consult a doctor before
embarking on any complementary therapy programme and on any matters relating to your
health, and in particular on any matters that may require diagnosis or medical attention.

A CIP catalogue record for this title is available from the
British Library and the Library of Congress

ISBN 978 1 84819 422 9
eISBN 978 0 85701 374 3

Printed and bound in United States by Integrated Books International.

Jessica Kingsley Publishers' policy is to use papers that are natural,
renewable and recyclable products and made from wood grown in
sustainable forests. The logging and manufacturing processes are expected
to conform to the environmental regulations of the country of origin.

Jessica Kingsley Publishers
Carmelite House
50 Victoria Embankment
London EC4Y 0DZ

www.singingdragon.com

For Stephanie
who helped me find my voice
in the excruciating silence

Contents

Preface

There is a Chinese idiom about a frog who lives at the bottom of a well who believes the sky to be a tiny blue dot, because that is all he can see in his narrow existence. Let us begin with the aspiration to have more awareness than the frog at the bottom of the well. The world of classical Chinese medicine is vast. If we want to understand, the first thing to do is climb out of our comfort zones.

This field guide is intended as a handbook to passages on clinical practice in the *Huángdì Nèijīng Sùwèn* 《黃帝內經素問》 The Yellow Emperor's Internal Classic, Plain Questions. It is meant to inspire and direct the reader to study the book in depth by engaging with the original text directly or through multiple translations. I believe this project will be of interest especially to practitioners in the field of Chinese medicine who are interested in classics. This book is meant to make the study of classical Chinese medicine a little less scary. If you've ever slogged through a passage (or a translation) thinking, "I'll never understand any of this!," this book is for you. If you've ever sat in (or walked out of) a class feeling frustrated, wondering, "Why do we have to study these ancient things anyway? I don't see how this relates...," this book is for you.

Every classics professor I've studied with emphasizes the importance of returning to the source material over and over again. A book that is only good the first time through is pulp fiction. A book that gives you more every time you return to it is a classic. However, there is no way that returning to a translation of a classic can measure up to returning to the original text. It is like reading Shakespeare translated into Mandarin. So much is lost in translation; no one version can ever hope to capture the definitive essence of the original. By its very nature, a translation is limited by the capacity of its translator, by both the limitations of their language proficiency and their comprehension of the subject matter.

It is for this reason that I have resisted the temptation to translate a classic of Chinese medicine into English. While I have the language skills, I do not think I have the clinical depth yet to do justice to my favorite classical texts. If we're looking at a purely academic or historical translation, others have done this already, most notably Paul Unschuld.* If you want an unabridged translation that is more affordable, I recommend Maoshing Ni.†

When I started this project in 2015, I had not yet read the *Sùwèn* in its entirety. I chose the *Huángdì Nèijīng* because it is the oldest extant text we have of classical Chinese medicine. I suspected from reading excerpts that it would vastly enrich my practice, and it has. There is an entire ocean of knowledge in here, of which I have managed to scoop up a teacupful. If your cup is empty, I shall pour what I have into your cup, to share what I have gleaned from the depths. Yet there is more here, so much more. Do not be daunted or discouraged at the start. There is no need to understand it all. There is no need to master everything. Even getting one line can yield substantial clinical results. Figure out what you are good at, and delve into that.

I am good at reading Chinese and writing English. I enjoy seeing patients and mentoring students, and I believe in the power of sharing. Some things, like love and wisdom, are increased and enriched when you hand them out. So, here is my tiny cup of

---

* Unschuld, P. (2011). *Huang Di Nei Jing Su Wen: An Annotated Translation of Huang Di's Inner Classic – Basic Questions: 2 volumes*. Berkeley, CA: University of California Press.

† Ni, M. (1995). *The Yellow Emperor's Classic of Medicine: A New Translation of the Neijing Suwen with Commentary*. Boston, MA: Shambhala.

insights into the incredibly rich world of an ancient healing art. Here you go. Enjoy.

Notes on the text

On the Chinese:

I use traditional characters, on the reasoning that simplified characters were not invented until the 1950s.

I use the archaic character (zhēn) 鍼 which means "acupuncture" in Japanese rather than the more modern (zhēn) 針 which means "needle". In most Chinese sources I find them used interchangeably.

I use (zhēn) 鍼 acupuncture needle and (cì) 刺 pricking instead of (zhēn) 針 needle/needling because (zhēn) 針 was originally a sewing needle. Japanese acupuncture has preserved the use of (zhēn) 鍼.

On Pinyin romanization:

I could not figure out how to type an umlaut ë in conjunction with tone marks, so all final umlaut ë appear as ē, é, ě, è.

I opted to pronounce "blood" as (xiě) 血, in colloquial Mandarin rather than the more formal and almost never used dictionary pronunciation (xuè). Blood is often colloquially pronounced as (xüě) with a third tone, but that pronunciation is not in the dictionary.

I opted to pronounce "cough" in its contemporary form, as (ké) 咳, rather than the formal (kài) 欬 because 欬 was an old form of writing the modern character.

On abbreviations:

The following abbreviations are used throughout this book.

Lu Lung

LI Large Intestine

St Stomach

Sp   Spleen

H   Heart

SI   Small Intestine

UB   Urinary Bladder

K   Kidney

P   Pericardium

SJ   Sanjiao

GB   Gallbladder

Lv   Liver

R   Ren

SHL: [line number] Shānghán Lùn
《傷寒論》 Discussion on Cold Damage

SW: [chapter number] Sùwèn
《素問》 Plain Questions

SWJZ Shuōwén Jiězì
《說文解字》 Explicating Words, Explaining Characters

Unschuld   Paul Unschuld's Huang Di Nei Jing Su Wen:
An Annotated Translation of Huang Di's Inner Classic – Basic
Questions

Wiseman   Pleco Chinese-English Dictionary App's version
of Nigel Wiseman's A Practical Dictionary of Chinese Medicine

On omissions:

Though this is not a line-by-line translation, I have made
every effort to create an overview of the text in its unabridged
entirety. If I omit a line or section on purpose, it is noted in the
footnotes.

A Brief History of the Text

Huángdì Nèijīng 《黃帝內經》 The Yellow Emperor's Internal Classic is first mentioned in the *Hàn Shū* 《漢書》 Book of Han compiled by historian Bān Gù 班固. Completed in 111, 19 years after Bān Gù's death in prison by his younger sister Bān Zhāo 班昭, the Book of Han mentions a number of medical classics, of which the *Huángdì Nèijīng* is the only one to survive intact.

Medical classics mentioned in the *Book of Han*

- *Huángdì Nèijīng* 《黃帝內經》 The Yellow Emperor's Internal Classic 18 volumes

- *Huángdì Wàijīng* 《黃帝外經》 The Yellow Emperor's External Classic 39 volumes

- *Biǎn Què Nèijīng* 《扁鵲內經》 Bian Que's Internal Classic 9 volumes

- *Biǎn Què Wàijīng* 《扁鵲外經》 Bian Que's External Classic 12 volumes

- *Bái Shì Nèijīng* 《白氏內經》 White Clan's Internal Classic 38 volumes

- *Bái Shì Wàijīng* 《白氏外經》 <u>White Clan's External Classic</u> 36 volumes

- *Bái Shì Pángpiān* 《白氏旁篇》 <u>White Clan's Side Articles</u> 25 volumes

Scholars of the *Huángdì Nèijīng* ascribe it to the late Warring States period (475–221 BC) because it contains so many parallels with 3rd Century BC Chinese literature. It is the oldest extant text on Chinese medicine, over 2000 years old.

The 4 great classics of Chinese medicine (zhōng yī sì dà jīng diǎn) 中醫四大經典

Huángdì Nèijīng 《黃帝內經》 *The Yellow Emperor's Internal Classic*	Also known as *Nèijīng* 《內經》	A book on fundamental Chinese medicine theory and acupuncture, compiled in the Warring States period (475–221 BC)
Huángdì Bāshíyī Nànjīng 《黃帝八十一難經》 *The Yellow Emperor's Classic of 81 Difficulties*	Also known as *Nànjīng* 《難經》	A 'study guide' of 81 difficulties found in the Nèijīng, compiled in the late Hàn Dynasty (ca. 25-220) that establishes clinical applications of 5 Element theory and pulse reading
Shénnóng Běncǎo Jīng 《神農本草經》 *Divine Husbandman's Materia Medica*	Also known as *Běnjīng* 《本經》	A compilation of 365 medicinal plants written down somewhere in the Qín/Hàn Dynasties (ca. 221 BC–220) but ascribed to Shénnóng 神農 "the Divine Husbandman," who lived around 2800 BC
Shānghán Zábìng Lùn 《傷寒雜病論》 *Discussion on Cold Damage and Miscellaneous Conditions*	Often split into: *Shānghán Lùn* 《傷寒論》 *Jīnguì Yào Lüè* 《金匱要略》	A collection of 269 herbal prescriptions with detailed diagnostic key signs, and symptoms written by physician Zhāng Zhòngjīng 張仲景 in the later Hàn Dynasty (ca. 206–220 BC)

In 762 BC, after 12 years' work, Táng Dynasty physician Wáng Bīng 王冰 published a revision of the first 9 volumes of the *Huángdì Nèijīng*, which he titled *Huángdì Nèijīng Sùwèn* 《黃帝內經素問》 <u>The Yellow Emperor's Internal Classic, Plain</u>

Questions. Eastern Hàn/Jìn Dynasty scholar Huángfǔ Mì 皇甫謐 (215–282), author of the *Zhēnjiǔ Jiǎyǐ Jīng* 《鍼灸甲乙經》 ABCs of Acupuncture and Moxibustion, first mentioned that the books called *Sùwèn* 《素問》 Plain Questions, and *Zhēnjīng* 《鍼經》 Needle Classic are the first and second of the 9 volumes of The Yellow Emperor's Internal Classic. Wáng Bīng's annotated edition of the *Sùwèn* confirmed Huángfǔ Mì's claim. Most scholars today agree that Needle Classic was an earlier title of the *Língshū* 《靈樞》 Magic Pivots, the second half of the *Huángdì Nèijīng*.

Wáng Bīng added 7 chapters to the *Sùwèn*, Chapters 66–71 and 74. He also added copious annotations in red ink, which are included in Paul Unschuld's translation. He listed Chapters 72 and 73 as lost, but Liú Wēnshū 劉溫舒 in the Sòng Dynasty (ca. 1098) claimed that they were only apocryphal, i.e. misplaced, and supplied text that some scholars believe he wrote himself.

This book includes in chronological order summaries of all 81 chapters ascribed to the *Huángdì Nèijīng* that comprise the *Sùwèn*, including those written by Wáng Bīng in the Tang Dynasty (ca. 762) and the Apocryphal Chapters 72 and 73 supplied by Liú Wēnshū in 1098.

Discussion on High Ancient Sky Truths

上古天真論

(shàng gǔ tiān zhēn lùn)

Chapter 1, Discussion on High Ancient Sky Truths, is about ideals. The first sentence introduces (huáng dì) 黃帝, the "Yellow Emperor." Huángdì is a title; his actual name, never directly mentioned in the text, is Gōngsūn Xuānyuán 公孫軒轅. The opening paragraph also sketches out briefly the ideal lifestory of a mythological ruler of ancient China: born with a god-like spirit and keen soul, well spoken by age 20, studied with many masters as a youth, grown to a manhood marked by (dūn mǐn) 敦敏 "groundedness and agility," finally completing his destiny by ascending to the immortal heavens.

Additionally, Xuānyuán 軒轅 is the name of a 17-star constellation, so perhaps the Emperor returned to the heavens where he belongs.

The first question the Emperor asks his (tiān shī) 天師 "Sky Master" is about aging and longevity. Tiānshī is also a title, possibly a rank; the Physician's actual name is Qí Bó 岐伯.

We hear him referred to by his name frequently throughout the *Nèijīng* 《內經》 <u>Internal Classic</u>.

The Emperor begins by asking Qi Bo, "Why is it that people used to live to 100 years old spry and vigorous, while nowadays people grow frail at merely 50?"[*] Qi Bo's answer describes the ideal lifestyle and philosophical outlook of a person who wishes to cultivate longevity. In short, those who live moderately in diet, exercise, sex, sleep, and emotions enjoy longer vigor.

Seven- and eight-year cycles of fertility

The second question the Emperor asks is about fertility. Qi Bo responds with the oft-quoted passage on the cycles of reproductive development and decline, which run every 7 years for females and every 8 years for males.[†] This is an essential passage for understanding menstruation and menopause, virility and aging.

♀ Age	Fertility
7	Kidney qi abundant, teeth change, hair grows
14	Tiānguǐ[1] and Chong[2] abundant, Ren[3] opens, menarche, therefore fertile
21	Kidney qi even, true teeth come in complete
28	Sinews and bones toughen, hair complete, body abundant and strong
35	Yangming weakens, face begins to dry, hair begins to fall
42	3 yang vessels weaken above, face totally dry, hair begins to whiten
49	Ren empty, Chong weak and scanty, Tiānguǐ runs out, menopause, therefore the body spoils i.e. becomes infertile

---

[*] 上古之人, 春秋皆度百歲而動作不衰, 今時之人, 年半百而動作皆衰者, 時世異耶？ (shàng gǔ zhī rén, chūn qiū jiē dù bǎi suì ér dòng zuò bù shuāi, jīn shí zhī rén, nián bàn bǎi ér dòng zuò jiē shuāi zhě, shí shì yì yé?).

[†] This also explains why girls develop faster than boys, and men age slower than women.

♂ Age	Fertility
8	Kidney qi solid, hair grows and teeth change
16	Kidney qi abundant, tiānguǐ arrives, essence qi overflows, yin yang harmonious, therefore fertile
24	Kidney qi even, sinews and bones powerful, therefore true teeth come in complete
32	Sinews and bones thriving and abundant, muscles full and strong
40	Kidney qi weakens, hair falls and teeth wither
48	Yang qi weakens and runs out above, face dry, hair and sideburns whiten
56	Liver qi weakens, sinews cannot move, tiānguǐ runs out, jīng-essence scanty, Kidney organ weak
64	Teeth and hair gone, 5 Zang weak, sinews and bones loose, tiānguǐ ends, therefore hair and sideburns white, body heavy, cannot walk straight, infertile

Four examples of exemplary living

Finally, the Emperor mentions four examples of exemplary living and their fantastic results, including the (zhēn rén) 真人 "true person," the (zhì rén) 至人 "ultimate person," and (shèng rén) 聖人 the "sage". We hear about the sage a lot more in subsequent chapters. The sage is an ideal of healthy living toward which people aspire, similar to Confucius' ideal (jūn zǐ) 君子 "gentleman."*

---

*   Confucius' "gentleman" is the same (jūn zǐ) 君子 as in (sì jūn zǐ tāng) 四君子 湯 Four Gentlemen's Decoction!

Big Discussion on Regulating Spirit in the Four Seasons

四氣調神大論

(sì qì tiáo shén dà lùn)

Chapter 2, Big Discussion on Regulating Spirit in the Four Seasons, is about seasons. Specifically, it describes the unique qualities of each season, sketches out a rubric for living in accordance with (sì qì) 四氣 the "four seasons," and what happens if we fail to (tiáo shén) 調神 "regulate spirit" to match the world. This is the chapter to read for lifestyle advice.

Dos and don'ts of the 4 seasons

	i.e.	Do	Do not	Consequences
Spring (chūn) 春	(fā chén) 發陳[4]	Sleep late, rise early Walk outdoors Let your hair down Wear loose clothing Create, give, reward	Kill, take, penalize	Harms Liver Becomes *Cold Changes* (hán biàn) 寒變 in summer
Summer (xià) 夏	(fán xiù) 蕃秀[5]	Sleep late, rise early Let buds come to fruit Let qi be released[6]	Get tired of the sun Be angry	Harms Heart Becomes *Intermittent Ague* (jiē nuè) 痎瘧 in autumn Get gravely ill in winter
Autumn (qiū) 秋	(róng píng) 容平[7]	Sleep early, rise early[8] Be calm[9] Withdraw shén-spirit and qi[10]		Harms Lung Get *Lienteric Diarrhea* (sūn xiè) 飧泄[11] in winter
Winter (dōng) 冬	(bì cáng) 閉藏[12]	Sleep early, rise late Wait for the sun to shine Be hidden/ concealed[13] Stay warm	Open the pores[14]	Harms Kidney Get *Atrophy Reversal* (wěi jué) 痿厥 in spring

The second paragraph uses the extended metaphor of an apocalyptic storm to further illustrate the detriments of going against the qi of each season. It tells us what will happen to the qi of each Zang if we counter the seasonal qi. I do not really understand how this passage relates to clinical practice, but I suspect it has something to do with the chronobiology explicated at length in *Sùwèn*, Chapters 66–74.

The merits of preventative medicine

The final paragraph states the merits of walking the Way of preventative medicine. It also contains a few useful analogies in favor of preventative medicine. I refer to this passage frequently when explaining to skeptical patients who feel as if acupuncture "does nothing" that their treatments are *preventing* bad things from happening. This was the first passage of the *Neijing* that I really felt I understood:

是故聖人不治已病治未病
(shì gù shèng rén bú zhì yǐ bìng zhì wèi bìng)
The sage treats disease not after but before it ever arises,

不治已亂治未亂, 此之謂也
(bú zhì yǐ luàn zhì wèi luàn, cǐ zhī wèi yě)
[and] governs* not after but before revolution arises.

夫病已成而後藥之
(fū bìng yǐ chéng ér hòu yào zhī)
To administer medicine after disease has taken hold

亂已成而後治之
(luàn yǐ chéng ér hòu zhì zhī)
To govern after revolution has taken hold

譬猶渴而穿井
(pì yóu kě ér chuān jǐng)
is like digging a well when thirsty

鬭而鑄錐
(dòu ér zhù zhuī)
[or] forging weapons when battle has already begun.

不亦晚乎
(bú yì wǎn hū)
That is to say, late!

---

*   The verb for treating disease and governing countries is the same one, (zhì) 治. The character originally meant to harness a river and keep it from flooding its banks; that is why it has a (shuǐ) 氵 water radical next to (tái) 台 platform.

Discussion on the Generation of Qi Through the Sky

生氣通天論

(shēng qì tōng tiān lùn)

Chapter 3, Discussion on the Generation of Qi Through the Sky, is about yang qi. Arguments for the heavy use of (fù zǐ) 附子 "aconite" in the Sìchuān Fire School tradition of herbs can be found in this chapter.

It begins with a paragraph about how (tiān qì) 天氣 "sky qi," i.e. weather, is reflected in the (yáng qì) 陽氣 of humans.

Four pathogenic factors that deplete yang qi

Pathogen	Signs and symptoms
Cold 寒 (hán)	Causes desires to transport and pivot, which disrupts biorhythms, thus shen and qi float
Heat 暑 (shǔ)	Sweat, vexations, panting, verbosity, body [feels] like embers, dispersed with sweat
Damp 濕 (shī)	Head feels wrapped,[15] damp-heat leads to big tendons cramp, small tendons atrophy
Qi 氣 (qì)	Swelling

Diseases and pathophysiology mentioned in Chapter 3

Disease	Pathophysiology
Boiling Reversal 煎厥 (jiān jué)	Vexation and labor exhaust jīng-essence, creating Aggregation (pǐ jī) 癖積 in summer
Thin Reversal 薄厥 (bó jué)	Fury exhausts form and qi, blood accumulates above
Asymmetrical Withering 偏枯 (piān kū)	Injured sinews, laxity and dysfunction, plus sweating on one side of the body
Acne Rash 痤痱 (cuó fèi)	Sweating meets damp
Foot Grows Large Boil 足生大疔 (zú shēng dà dīng)	[Ingesting] thick [flavors] and alcohol
Pimples 皶 (zhā)	Exertion/Sweating in wind, wearing too little in cold
Acne 痤 (cuó)	[Emotional] repression
Hunchback 大僂 (dà lóu)	Cold qi follows and sinks into vessels, flesh and interstices
Shock Terrors 驚駭 (jīng hài)	Back-shū qi transforms thinly into paranoia
Carbuncle Swelling 癰腫 (yōng zhǒng)	Yíng-nutritive qi not following and counterflow into flesh and interstices
Wind Ague 風瘧 (fēng nuè)	Pò sweat incomplete, form weak and qi flickering, acupoints shut

Sun cycle of yang qi actions

平旦人氣生
(píng dàn rén qì shēng)
At dawn, human qi is born.

日中而陽氣隆
(rì zhōng ér yáng qì lóng)
At noon, yang qi swells.

日西而陽氣已虛
(rì xī ér yáng qì yǐ xū)
When the sun slants west, yang qi has become deficient,

氣門乃閉
(qì mén nǎi bì)
the qi gates close.

是故暮而收拒
(shì gù mù ér shōu jù)
Therefore at dusk withdraw,

無擾筋骨
(wú rǎo jīn gǔ)
do not disturb sinew and bone,

無見霧露
(wú jiàn wù lù)
do not expose to fog and dew.

Qi Bo also speaks of the relationship between yin and yang, and the consequences of yin-yang imbalance. Then the chapter goes back to pathophysiology of disorders related to yang qi.

Diseases and pathophysiology mentioned in Chapter 3 continued...

More diseases!	Pathophysiology
Hemorrhoids 痔 (zhì)	Overeating leads to separation of sinews and vessels, leads to diarrhea
Qi Counterflow 氣逆 (qì nì)	Overdrinking [of alcohol]
High Bone Ruin 高骨乃壞 (gāo gǔ nǎi huài)	Heavy lifting leads to damaging of Kidney qi
Cold Heat 寒熱 (hán rè)	Exposure to wind
Grotto Diarrhea 洞泄 (dòng xiè)	Damage by wind in spring leads to lingering pathogens
Intermittent Ague 痎瘧 (jiē nuè)	Damage by heat in summer
Atrophy Reversal 痿厥 (wěi jué)	Damage by damp in autumn leads to upward counterflow and cough
Warm Disease 溫病 (wēn bìng)	Damage by cold in winter

Discussion on True Words from the Golden Cabinet

金匱真言論

(jīn guì zhēn yán lùn)

Chapter 4, Discussion on True Words from the Golden Cabinet,* introduces the concept of (wǔ xíng) 五行 "five elements," also known as the five phases. It covers which seasons triumph over† which, where disease is located, and what types of disorders are likely.

---

* The same (jīn guì) 金匱 as in (*Jīn Guì Yào Luè*) 《金匱要略》 Essentials from the Golden Cabinet.

† 勝 (shèng): to win, defeat, triumph over, get the better of. This is the verb that the Sùwèn uses for the overacting/controlling cycle.

Controlling cycle: Five winds

The Emperor asks, "Sky has eight winds.* Jīng-channels have five winds. What does this mean?"

Qi Bo answers, "Eight winds express pathogens, which become jīng-channel wind. [If they] reach the five Zang, pathogenic qi creates disease." He states the controlling cycle in terms of seasons (i.e. Spring triumphs over longsummer. Longsummer triumphs over winter. Winter triumphs over summer. Summer triumphs over autumn. Autumn triumphs over spring).

~ Wind	Born by	Ill at	Acupoints[16] at	Location	Signs and symptoms
East	Spring	Liver	Neck/Nape	Head	*Nasal Congestion* 鼽 (qiú) *Nosebleed* 衄 (nǜ)
South	Summer	Heart	Chest/Ribs	Zang	[Occur at] Chest and Ribs
West	Autumn	Lung	Shoulders/Back	Shoulders and Back[17]	*Wind Ague* 風瘧 (fēng nüè)
North	Winter	Kidney	Lumbar/ Buttocks	4 limbs	*Impediment* 痹 (bì) *Reversal* 厥 (jué)
Center[18]	Earth	Spleen	Spine	N/A	*Grotto Diarrhea* 洞泄 (dòng xiè) *Cold Strike* 寒中 (hán zhōng)

---

*   **Acu Trivia!** 八風 (bā fēng): "8 Winds" is the name of a set of acupoints in the webbing between the toes.

Yin yang aspects of the sun cycle and how it is reflected in humans

	Yang within yang	Yin within yang	Yin within yin	Yang within yin
Day	Dawn to Noon	Noon to Dusk	Dusk to Midnight	Midnight to Dawn
Human	Back: Heart	Back: Lung	Abdomen: Kidney	Abdomen: Liver

Yin yang location and season of disease

	Human	Body	Organs	Disease
Yin	Internal	Back	Zang	Winter/Autumn
Yang	External	Abdomen	Fu	Summer/Spring

The five Zang reflect the four seasons

Then the Emperor asks if the five Zang reflect the four seasons, and Qi Bo answers, "Yes." Qi Bo then lists each direction's corresponding color, which Zang it enters, which orifice it opens at, where it stores jīng-essence, what disease it expresses, and its corresponding: flavor, element,* livestock, grain, resonating star, body part where disease commonly occurs, sound, number, and scent.

Direction	East	South	Center	West	North
Color	Blue-Green	Red	Yellow	White	Black
Enters[19]	Liver	Heart	Spleen	Lung	Kidney
Orifice	Eye	Ear	Mouth	Nose	2 yin[20]
Disease location	Head	Zang	Tongue base	Back	4 limbs
Flavor	Sour	Bitter	Sweet	Spicy	Salty
Category*	Grass and Wood	Fire	Earth	Metal	Water

---

* The character used here is (lèi) 類 which means "category."

Livestock	Chicken	Goat	Ox	Horse	Pig
Grain	Wheat	Sticky millet[21]	Millet	Rice	Bean
Star	Jupiter	Mars	Saturn	Venus	Mercury
Condition[22] at	Sinews	Vessels	Flesh	Skin[23]	Bone
Music[24]	Mi	So	Do	Re	La
Number	8	7	5	9	6
Scent	Rank	Scorched	Fragrant	Fishy	Rotten

At the end of Chapter 4, Qi Bo emphasizes that those who are good at taking pulse carefully observe the counterflow and following of the five Zang and six Fu, the yin-yang of exterior and interior, the order of female and male, the heart's intention combined with jīng-essence. He adds an admonishment against teaching the wrong person or imparting the wrong truth.

Big Discussion on Yin Yang Reflection Images

陰陽應象大論

(yīn yáng yìng xiàng dà lùn)

Chapter 5, Big Discussion on Yin Yang Reflection Images, is about how yin and yang (yìng xiàng) 應象 "reflects things" in the body and the world. More specifically, it goes into (qì) 氣 and (xíng) 形 "form," (qīng) 清 "clear" and (zhuó) 濁 "turbid," (hán) 寒 "cold" and (rè) 熱 "heat."

Yin yang: definitions and functions

The Emperor states:

陰陽者, 天地之道也
(yīn yáng zhě, tiān dì zhī dào yě)
Yin and yang are the Way of sky and land,

萬物之綱紀
(wàn wù zhī gāng jì)
The outline and record of ten thousand things,

變化之父母

(biàn huà zhī fù mǔ)

The father and mother of change and transformation,

生殺之本始

(shēng shā zhī běn shǐ)

The root and beginning of birth and killing,

神明之府也

(shén míng zhī fǔ yě)

The mansion of spirit and brightness,

治病必求於本

(zhì bìng bì qiú yú běn)

To treat disease [one] must beg of the root [cause].

故積陽為天, 積陰為地

(gù jī yáng wéi tiān, jī yīn wéi dì)

Thus, accumulating yang becomes sky, accumulating yin becomes land.

陰靜陽躁, 陽生陰長, 陽殺陰藏

(yīn jìng yáng zào, yáng shēng yīn zhǎng, yáng shā yīn cáng)

Yin is quiet. Yang is restless. Yang begets. Yin grows. Yang kills. Yin hides.

陽化氣, 陰成形

(yáng huà qì, yīn chéng xíng)

Yang transforms qi. Yin creates form.

寒氣生濁, 熱氣生清

(hán qì shēng zhuó, rè qì shēng qīng)

Cold qi creates turbid. Hot qi creates clear.

清氣在下, 則生飧泄

(qīng qì zài xià, zé shēng sūn xiè)

Clear qi below creates *Lienteric Diarrhea*.

濁氣在上, 則生䐜脹
(zhuó qì zài shàng, zé shēng chēn zhàng)
Turbid qi above creates creates *Bloating Distension*.

此陰陽反作, 病之逆從也
(cǐ yīn yáng fǎn zuò, bìng zhī nì cóng yě)
This is the flip side of yin and yang, the counterflow and following of disease.

We also learn about clear yang and turbid yin, water and fire, qi and flavor, the alchemy of digestion and its effects of qi transformation, external pathogenic factors versus internal emotional factors. Since this is a summary for clinical relevance, and not a translation, I will resist the temptation to go through it all line by line, but I find the following lines pertinent to orthopedic diagnosis.

Basic orthopedic diagnosis

寒傷形, 熱傷氣
(hán shāng xíng, rè shāng qì)
Cold harms form. Heat harms qi.

氣傷痛, 形傷腫
(qì shāng tòng, xíng shāng zhǒng)
Injured qi is painful. Injured form is swollen.

故先痛而後腫者, 氣傷形也
(gù xiān tòng ér hòu zhǒng zhě, qì shāng xíng yě)
Therefore, first painful and then swollen, [it is because] qi has harmed the form.

先腫而後痛者, 形傷氣也
(xiān zhǒng ér hòu tòng zhě, xíng shāng qì yě)
First swollen then painful, [it means] form has harmed the qi.

Generating cycle

We are then introduced to the generating cycle, which is much more complex than the version I learned in acupuncture school.

	East	South	Center	West	North
Generates	Wind	Heat	Damp	Dry	Cold
Generates	Wood	Fire	Earth	Metal	Water
Generates	Sour	Bitter	Sweet	Spicy	Salty
Generates	Liver	Heart	Spleen	Lung	Kidney
Generates	Sinew	Blood	Flesh	Skin	Bone
Generates	Heart	Spleen	Lung	Kidney	Liver
~ governs ~	Liver/Eye[25]	Heart/Tongue	Spleen/Mouth	Lung/Nose	Kidney/Ear
Weather	Wind	Heat	Damp	Dry	Cold
Land	Wood	Fire	Earth	Metal	Water
Body	Sinew	Vessels	Flesh	Skin	Bone
Zang	Liver	Heart	Spleen	Lung	Kidney
Color	Blue-green	Red	Yellow	White	Black
Music	Mi	So	Do	Re	La
Sound	Shout	Laugh	Sing	Weep	Moan
Change	Grip	Worry	Belch	Cough	Shiver
Orifice	Eye	Tongue	Mouth	Nose	Ear
Flavor	Sour	Bitter	Sweet	Spicy	Salty

Controlling cycle

Then we are introduced to the controlling cycle, which is pretty much the same as what we learn in school, with a few unexpected relationships which I have highlighted in **bold**.

~ harms ~	Anger/ Liver	Joy/Heart	Thought/ Spleen	**Worry/** Lung	Fear/ Kidney
~ overrides ~	Sadness/ Anger	Fear/Joy	Anger/ Thought	Joy/**Worry**	Thought/ Fear
~ harms ~	Wind/ Sinews	Heat/Qi	Damp/ Flesh	**Heat**/Skin	Cold/ Blood
~ overrides ~	Dry/Wind	Cold/Heat	Wind/ Damp	Cold/Heat	**Dry**/Cold
~ harms ~	Sour/ Sinews	Bitter/Qi	Sweet/ Flesh	Spicy/Skin	Salty/ Blood
~ overrides ~	Spicy/Sour	Salty/ Bitter	Sour/Sweet	Bitter/ Spicy	Sweet/ Salty

The Emperor asks about imbalances of yin and yang and Qi Bo gives general examples. Then the Emperor asks about regulating yin and yang and Qi Bo reiterates aging (without really going into specifics about how). The seven harms and eight benefits are mentioned but not explained. Those who know it are strong; those who do not grow old.

Another thing I find interesting in this chapter is the explanation for why most people are right-handed. Apparently, sky is insufficient in the northwest, and land* is not full in the southeast. This means that yang gathers above in the left side of the body (assuming the sage is standing facing south) and yin collects in the lower parts on the right side of the body, making the right arm and leg more adept and the left ear and eye more keen. Also, climatic energies are reflected in the body as follows:

Qi of	Passes through
Weather	Lung
Land	Esophagus
Thunder	Liver
Grain	Spleen
Rain	Kidney

---

* By "land" I mean (dì) 地 versus (tǔ) 土 "earth."

The conclusion is long and packed with information on diagnosis and treatment principles, so I will just pick out my favorite lines:

故善治者治皮毛
(gù shàn zhì zhě zhì pí máo)
Therefore those adept at treatment treat [disease at] the skin and pores,

其次治肌膚
(qí cì zhì jī fū)
those less adept treat [disease at] the muscles and fascia,*

其次治筋脈
(qí cì zhì jīn mài)
those less adept treat [disease at] the sinews and vessels,

其次治六府
(qí cì zhì liù fǔ)
those less adept treat [disease at] the six Fu,

其次治五藏
(qí cì zhì wǔ zàng)
those less adept treat [disease at] the five Zang.

治五藏者, 半死半生也
(zhì wǔ zàng zhě, bàn sǐ bàn shēng yě)
Treating [disease at] the five Zang, half die and half live.

故天之邪氣, 感則害人五藏
(gù tiān zhī xié qì, gǎn zé hài rén wǔ zàng)
Therefore the pathogenic qi of weather harms the five Zang.

水穀之寒熱, 感則害於六府
(shuǐ gǔ zhī hán rè, gǎn zé hài yú liù fǔ)
The temperature of food and water harms the six Fu.

地之濕氣, 感則害皮肉筋脈
(dì zhī shī qì, gǎn zé hài pí ròu jīn mài)

---

* In these two lines, I think (pí máo) 皮毛 indicates exterior surface and (jī fū) 肌膚 indicates internal surface, i.e. fascia just below the skin.

The damp qi of geography harms skin, flesh, sinews and vessels.

故善用鍼者, 從陰引陽, 從陽引陰
(gù shàn yòng zhēn zhě, cóng yīn yǐn yáng, cóng yáng yǐn yīn)
Therefore those adept at acupuncture guide yin to yang, guide yang to yin,

以右治左, 以左治右
(yǐ yòu zhì zuǒ, yǐ zuǒ zhì yòu)
treat left with right, treat right with left,

以我知彼, 以表知裡
(yǐ wǒ zhī bǐ, yǐ biǎo zhī lǐ)
know the other through the self, know the interior through the exterior,

以觀過與不及之理, 見微得過
(yǐ guān guò yǔ bù jí zhī lǐ, jiàn wēi dé guò)
from observing the minutiae of excess and insufficiencies,

用之不殆
(yòng zhī bú dài)
use [skills] without peril.

Discussion on the Separation and Convergence of Yin and Yang

陰陽離合論

(yīn yáng lí hé lùn)

Chapter 6, Discussion on the Separation and Convergence of Yin and Yang, is much shorter than Chapter 5. It is a follow-up conversation after the great lecture Qi Bo gives on how yin and yang are reflected in all things.

The Emperor states, "I understand sky is yang, land is yin, sun is yang, moon is yin, and humans reflect the great and small months and 365 days, but I do not understand how 3 yin and 3 yang fit in."

Qi Bo answers rather cryptically with yet another explanation of yin and yang, "It is fractal-like, with countless examples, yet adheres to one principle. The sprout that has not come out of the ground is yin within yin; the sprout that has come out is yang within yin. Yang motivates the seasonal actions of birth, growth, harvest, and hibernation. This can also be counted in humans."

The Emperor says he is willing to hear about the separation and union of yin and yang.*

Qi Bo then describes the six channels and their entry points.

Six channels and entry points

	Location	Begins	~ within Yin	Action
太陽 Tàiyáng	Above Shaoyin[26]	至陰 (zhì yīn) UB67[27]	Yang	Open
陽明 Yángmíng	Before Taiyin[28]	歷兌 (lì duì) St45	Yang	Close
少陽 Shàoyáng	Exterior of Jueyin	竅陰 (qiào yīn) GB44	Lesser yang	Hinge
太陰 Tàiyīn	Center of Yin[29]	隱白 (yǐn bái) Sp1	Yin	Open
少陰 Shàoyīn	Behind Taiyin	湧泉 (yǒng quán) K1	Lesser yin	Hinge
厥陰 Juéyīn	In front of Shaoyin	大敦 (dà dūn) Lv1	Ending[30] yin	Close

There are a few lines here I do not fully grasp. Taiyang, Yangming, and Shaoyang make one yang by a...texture? called (bó ér wù fú) 博而勿浮. Taiyin, Shaoyin, and Jueyin make one yin called (bó ér wù chén) 博而勿沈. I think these are pulse images, maybe, because (fú) 浮 is "floating" and (chén) 沈 is "sinking," i.e. deep. When yin and yang accumulate and spread over the course of a week, the qi inside and form outside do something mutual called (xiāng chéng) 相成—they complete each other(?).

---

* Huangdi often says (yuàn wén) 願聞 "[I am] willing to hear" when he is asking a question; I find this a charming format to indicate both his dignity and humbleness.

Addendum on Yin and Yang

陰陽別論

(yīn yáng bié lùn)

Chapter 7, Addendum on Yin and Yang, is about the yin and yang of pulse reading.

The Emperor asks about the 4 (jīng) 經 and 12 (cóng) 從. I am not sure if jīng here refers to meridians (why are there only 4?); cóng as a character means "following [the flow]" so maybe the 4 jīng here refers to the 4 Extraordinary Vessels (Chōng, Rèn, Dū, Dài) and the 12 cóng refers to the 12 Organ Meridians proper, which developmentally "follow" the 4 extraordinary vessels.

Anyway, Qi Bo tells the Emperor that the 4 jīng reflect the 4 seasons, the 12 cóng reflect the 12 months, and the 12 months reflect the 12 (mài) 脈. Again, I am not sure if mài here means "pulses" or "vessels."

Qi Bo adds, "Those who know yang know yin, those who know yin know yang. Each yang has 5, for 5 times 5 equals 25 yang. That which we call yin is the true Zang; if you see it, it is defeated. If it is defeated, [the patient] must die. That which we call yang is the yang of the stomach and digestion.* Differentiating yang tells us the disease location; differentiating yin tells us the date of mortality. The three yang are at the head. The three yin are at the hand. This is known as one."

Attributes of yin and yang

~ Pulse	Liver	Heart	Lung	Kidney	Spleen
Die in ~ days	18	9	23	7	4

Death prognoses

Yin	Leaving	Quiet	Late
Yang	Arriving	Active	Rapid

Diseases mentioned in Chapter 7

Disease of	Signs and symptoms	Spreads to become
2 yang	*Express [in] Heart/Spleen* 發心脾 (fā xīn pí) *Limited Flexion/Extension* 不得引曲 (bù dé yǐn qǔ) *Amenorrhea* 女子不月 (nǚ zǐ bú yuè)	*Wind Wasting* 風消 (fēng xiāo) *Breath Sprint*[31] 息賁 (xī bēn)
3 yang	*Cold Heat* 寒熱 (hán rè) *Carbuncle Swelling*[32] 癰腫 (yōng zhǒng) *Atrophy Reversal with Calf Weakness* 痿厥腨痛 (wěi júe chuǎi yuān)	*Rope Marsh* 索澤 (suǒ zé) *Genital Hernia* 穨疝 (tuí shàn)

---

* 胃脘 (weì wǎn): stomach and...digestive cavities? (e.g. R13 = 上脘 (shàng wǎn) upper wan, R12 = 中脘 (zhōng wǎn) central wan, R10 = 下脘 (xià wǎn) lower wan).

1 yang	*Scant Qi* 少氣 (shǎo qì) *Tendency for Cough* 善欬 (shàn ké) *Tendency for Diarrhea* 善泄 (shàn xiè)	*Heart Pull* 心掣 (xīn chè) *Block*, i.e. continuous vomiting 隔 (gé)
2 yang + 1 yin	*Shock Terrors* 驚駭 (jīng hài) *[Upper] Back Pain* 背痛 (bèi tòng) *Tendency for Hiccups* 善噫 (shàn yī) *Tendency for Yawns* 善欠 (shàn qiàn) This is called *Wind Reversal* 風厥 (fēng jué)	
2 yin + 1 yang	*Tendency for Distension* 善脹 (shàn zhàng) *Heart Fullness* 心滿 (xīn mǎn) *Tendency for Flatulence* 善氣 (shàn qì)	
3 yang + 3 yin	*Asymmetrical Withering*, aka hemiplegia 偏枯 (piān kū) *Atrophy Easily* 痿易 (wěi yì) *Inability to Lift the Limbs* 四肢不舉 (sì zhī bù jǔ)	

Pulse textures in Chapter 7

鉤 (gōu) "Hook"	1 yang
毛 (máo) "Feather"	1 yin
絃 (xián) "Wiry"	Yang excessive and rushed
石 (shí) "Stone"	Yang arrives and ends
溜 (liū) "Slide"	Yin and yang mutual excess

The emphasis of this chapter seems to be the interpretation of extreme pulses and their corresponding conditions.

Extreme pulses: dead yin, live yang, duplicate yin, pì yin

	Lung of Heart	Heart of Liver	Kidney of Lung	Spleen of Kidney
Is known as	Dead yin	Live yang	Duplicate yin	Pì yin[33]
Die in ~ days	3	4	N/A	N/A

Extreme pulses: signs and symptoms, prognoses, disease names

Pulse	Symptoms/Prognosis	Disease name
Knotted yang	Swollen limbs	
Knotted yin	Hematochezia*	
Yin > yang	Lower abdomen swollen	*Stone Water* 石水 (shí shuǐ)
2 yang knotted		*Wasting* 消 (xiāo)
3 yang knotted		*Block*, i.e. continuous vomiting 隔 (gé)
3 yin knotted		*Water* 水 (shuǐ)
1 yin + 1 yang		*Throat Impediment* 喉痹 (hóu bì)
Yin strike yang separate		*Pregnancy* 有子 (yǒu zǐ)
Yin yang deficient		*Intestinal Blockage* 腸癖 (cháng pǐ)
Yang added to yin		*Sweat* 汗 (hàn)
Yin xu yang strike		*Avalanche Menorrhagia* 崩 (bēng)
3 yin all strike	Die in 20 days at midnight	
2 yin all strike	Die in 13 days at dusk	
1 yin all strike	Die in 10 days	
3 yang all strike and gǔ	Die in 3 days	
3 yang 3 yin all strike	Heart and abdomen full, limited extension/flexion, die in 5 days	
2 yang all strike	Disease is warm, fatal die within 10 days	

---

*   Defecate blood volume one 升 (shēng) ~200ml, more knotted, two 升 (shēng) 400ml; more knotted three 升 (shēng) 600ml.

Discussion on the Secret Code of Soul Orchid

靈蘭秘典論

(líng lán mì diǎn lùn)

Chapter 8, Discussion on the Secret Code of Soul Orchid, is an extended metaphor of the body as government, which assigns each of the 12 organs an official position. "Secret Code of Soul Orchid" sounds like a video game, but actually refers to 靈臺 (líng tái) "Soul Bier,"* an observatory for looking at the stars, and 蘭室 (lán shì) "Orchid Chamber," the Emperor's Imperial Library.

The Emperor says, "I am willing to hear about the offices and duties of the 12 organs and their [social] class."

Qi Bo answers, "What an excellent question! Let me explain."

---

* 靈臺 (líng tái): Soul Bier, an observatory for looking at the stars, also a bier for ancestral worship or funerals. King Wen of the Zhou Dynasty built one in today's Shaanxi Province. **Acu Trivia!** (líng tái) 靈臺 is the name of Du10.

Official duties of the 12 organs

Organ	Official of ~ 之官 (zhī guān)	Duties (~ are exuded by it) ~ 出焉 (chū yān)
Heart	Emperor 君主 (jūn zhǔ)	Spirit and brightness 神明 (shén míng)
Lung	Minister 相傅 (xiāng fù)	Governance and (jié) 節[34] 治節 (zhì jié)
Liver	General 將軍 (jiāng jūn)	Strategy and deliberation 謀慮 (móu lǜ)
Gallbladder	Justice 中正 (zhōng zhèng)	Judgment and decisions 決斷 (jué duàn)
Pericardium[35]	Jester 臣使 (chén shǐ)	Joy and music 喜樂 (xǐ lè)
Spleen and Stomach	Granary 倉廩 (cāng lǐn)	Five flavors 五味 (wǔ wèi)
Large Intestine	Passkeeper 傳道 (chuán dào)	Change and transformation 變化 (biàn huà)
Small Intestine	Sorter 受盛 (shòu chéng)	Transforming substance 化物 (huà wù)
Kidney	Strengthener 做強 (zuò qiáng)	Talent and agility 伎巧 (jì qiǎo)
Sānjiāo	Irrigation 決瀆 (jué dú)	Waterways 水道 (shuǐ dào)
Bladder	Wetlands 州都 (zhōu dū)	Stores fluids, qi transformation for exudation 「津液藏焉, 氣化則能出矣」 (jīn yè cáng yān, qì huà zé néng chū yǐ)

The rest of the chapter is Qi Bo giving the Emperor allegorical advice on the hierarchical chain reactions of good government which may be applied to preventative health care. The Emperor ends the chapter by stating that he will choose an auspicious date to store this precious information in his library, the Chamber of Soul Orchids.*

---

* 靈蘭之室 (líng lán zhī shì): Chamber of Soul Orchids.

Discussion on the Six Nodes and Organ Images

六節藏象論

(liù jié zàng xiàng lùn)

Chapter 9, Discussion on the Six Nodes and Organ Images, is about the numerology of sky and land as related to humans. It contains some definitions of time that must be significant, because when the Emperor asks, "What is qi?* Please relieve this confusion for me!" Qi Bo demurs for the first time since his Emperor started asking him questions, "This is a secret from an ancient emperor† passed down to me by my late teacher."

The Emperor politely insists, "Please, allow me to hear [it]."

---

* Like the title of Chapter 2, this qi refers to a span of time. Four qi in Chapter 2 refers to the four seasons, and six qi in Chapter 9 refers to 15-day Solar Terms.

† 上帝 (shàng dì): literally "high emperor."

Definitions of time: rì, hòu, qì, shí, qì yín, qì pò

5 (rì) 日 days[36] = (hòu) 候 wait[37]	
3 (hòu) 候 waits = (qì) 氣 solar term	
6 (qì) 氣 solar terms = (shí) 時 season	
4 (shí) 時 seasons = (suì) 歲 year	

Qi Bo also gives us the controlling cycle of the seasons again, using "longsummer" for earth (see Appendix A), and tells us that the overacting of arriving before the proper time is called (qì yín) 氣淫 "qi excess." The deficiency of not arriving by the proper time is called (qì pò) 氣迫 "qi oppressed."

Organ images

The Emperor then asks, "What are organ images?" and Qi Bo answers:

	Root		Luster	Filled at	~ within ~	Goes through ~ qi
Heart	Birth	Change of Shén 神	Face	Vessels	Taiyang/ Yang	Summer (xià) 夏
Lung	Qi	Place of Pò 魄	Pores	Skin	Taiyin/ Yang	Autumn (qiū) 秋
Kidney	Seal[38]	Place of Jīng 精	Hair	Bone	Shaoyin/ Yin	Winter (dōng) 冬
Liver	Final	Dwelling of Hún 魂	Nails	Sinew[39]	Shaoyang/ Yang	Spring (chūn) 春
Spleen[40]	Granary	Dwelling of Yíng 營	Lips[41]	Muscle	Ultimate Yin[42]	Earth (tǔ) 土

Qi Bo adds, "Gallbladder makes decisions for all 11 organs."*

---

* 「凡十一藏取決於膽也。」 (fán shí yī zàng qǔ jué yú dǎn yě).

Disease location diagnosis: carotid versus radial pulse

Number of times larger than normal	At	Illness at/is called
1	Carotid pulse	Shaoyang
2		Taiyang
3		Yangming
4+		Repelled yang (gé yáng) 格陽
1	Radial pulse	Jueyin
2		Shaoyin
3		Taiyin
4+		Blocked yin (guān yīn) 關陰
4+	Both carotid and radial pulses	Block and repulsion (guān gé) 關格[43]

On the Generation and Completion of the Five Zang

五藏生成

(wǔ zàng shēng chéng)

Chapter 10 has no frame at all; it is pure lecture, On the Generation* and Completion of the Five Zang. As such, the content is best organized into tables.

---

* 生 (shēng): to generate, to create, birth, life, raw (as in shēng dì huáng 生地黃), etc.

Five elements: convergence, glory, master

	合 (hé) Convergence	榮 (róng) Glory	主 (zhǔ) Mastered by
心 (xīn) Heart	脈 (mài) Vessels	色 (sè) Complexion	腎 (shèn) Kidney
肺 (fèi) Lung	皮 (pí) Skin	毛 (máo) Body hair	心 (xīn) Heart
肝 (gān) Liver	筋 (jīn) Sinews	爪 (zhǎo) Nails	肺 (fèi) Lung
脾 (pí) Spleen	肉 (ròu) Flesh	唇 (chún) Lips	肝 (gān) Liver
腎 (shèn) Kidney	骨 (gǔ) Bone	髮 (fà) Hair	脾 (pí) Spleen

Five flavors of injury

Overeat	Consequences
Salty	Vessels coagulate and change color
Bitter	Skin withers and body hair uproots
Spicy	Sinews cramp and nails dry
Sour	Flesh wrinkles/calluses and lips chap
Sweet	Bones hurt and hair falls out

Five flavors of convergence

Organ	Desired flavor
Heart	Bitter
Lung	Spicy
Liver	Sour
Spleen	Sweet
Kidney	Salty

Five Zangs' qi: complexions of death and life

Complexion	Color of death	Color of life
Green	Grass shoots	Kingfisher feather
Yellow	Zhǐ shí*	Crab belly
Black	Altar soot	Raven feather
Red	Clotted blood	Rooster wattles
White	Dry bone	Boar fat

Five Zang-generated external glory

[When] born of	Is like silk wrapping
Heart	Cinnabar
Lung	Vermillion
Liver	Burgundy/Violet
Spleen	Guā lóu shí†
Kidney	Purple

Five Zangs' complexion/flavor

Complexion	Zang	Flavor
White	Lung	Spicy
Red	Heart	Bitter
Green	Liver	Sour
Yellow	Spleen	Sweet
Black	Kidney	Salty

---

* 枳實 (zhǐ shí) "immature bitter orange."

† 瓜蔞實 (guā lóu shí) "trichosanthes fruit."

Five colors/body parts

Color	Body part
Red	Vessel
White	Skin
Green	Sinew
Yellow	Flesh
Black	Bone

The dawn and dusk of four limbs and eight streams

All	Belong to
Vessels	Eye
Marrow	Brain
Sinews	Joints
Blood	Heart
Qi	Lung

When we sleep, blood returns to liver

~ receives blood	And can
Liver	See
Feet	Walk
Hands	Grip
Fingers	Pinch

If we sleep in the wind, blood coagulates in ~ and becomes ~

Surface 膚 (fū)	*Impediment* 痹 (bì)
Vessels 脈 (mài)	*Coagulation* 泣 (qì)
Leg 足 (zú)	*Reversal* 厥 (jué)

Humans have 12 big valleys, 354 small streams, minus 12 acupoints,* all of which defensive qi lingers and stops at, places where evil qi guests. Needle or stone the source to dispel.

Diseases mentioned in Chapter 10

Signs and symptoms	Diagnosis	Correction needed at
Headache 頭痛 (tóu tòng) *Vertex Disease* 巔疾 (diān jí)	Deficient below, excess above	Foot Shaoyin[44]
Sudden Dizziness 徇蒙 (xùn mēng) *Head Shaking* 招尤 (zhāo yóu) *Blurry Vision* 目冥 (mù míng) *Deafness* 耳聾 (ěr lóng)	Excess below, deficient above	Foot Shaoyang[45]
Abdominal Distension 腹脹 (fù zhàng)	Reversal below, veiling above	Foot Taiyin/Yangming
Cough 欬 (ké) *Panting* 喘 (chuǎn)	Reversal in chest/center	Hand Yangming/Taiyin
Heart Vexation 心煩 (xīn fán) *Headache* 頭痛 (tóu tòng)	Disease in diaphragm/center	Hand Juyang/Shaoyin

---

* 少十二俞 (shǎo shí èr shū): I am not sure if this means "minus" 12 acupoints, or 12 "young(er)" acupoints. The text does not specify which 12 acupoints it is referring to.

Pulse presentations for Qi accumulation

Pulse	Qi accumulation in	Presentation	Etiology	Disease
Red[46]	Middle	Sometimes harmed by food?	Exterior invasion due to Heart deficiency from thought and worry	*Heart Impediment* 心痹 (xīn bì)
White[47]	Chest	Shock Deficient asthma	Sex while intoxicated	*Lung Impediment*[48] 肺痹 (fèi bì)
Green[49]	Epigastrium/ Flank	Low back pain Cold feet Headache	Cold damp, same as *Hernia*	*Liver Impediment* 肝痹 (gān bì)
Yellow[50]	Abdomen	Qi reversal	Wind on 4 limbs while sweating	*Reversal Hernia*[51] 厥疝 (jué shàn)
Black[52]	Hypogastrium	N/A	Sleeping after bathing in clear water	*Kidney Impediment* 肾痹 (shèn bì)

Five complexions of Extraordinary Vessels

Live		Die	
Face	Eye	Face	Eye
Yellow	Green	Green	Red
Yellow	Red	Red	White
Yellow	White	Green	Black
Yellow	Black	Black	White
		Red	Green

Addendum on the Five Zang

五藏別論

(wǔ zàng bié lùn)

Chapter 11, Addendum on the Five Zang, is about the extraordinary organs, and the difference between (mǎn) 滿 "full" and (shí) 實 "solid."*

First, the Emperor asks about physicians who consider brain and marrow to be Zang, or the stomach and intestines to be Zang.

Definitions: extraordinary Fu-organs and transformational Fu-organs, Gate of Po

Qi Bo answers, "Brain, marrow, bone, vessels, gallbladder, uterus, these six are created by land qi, stored in yin and reflecting land, therefore they store and do not release and are known as (qí

---

* 滿 (mǎn): full [of energy] versus 實 (shí): solid [with tangible substance]. This is the same character 實 from 8 principles diagnosis; pathologically, (shí) 實 means excess/replete and (xū) 虛 means deficient/vacuous.

héng zhī fǔ) 奇恆之府 'the extraordinary Fu-organs.' Stomach, large intestine, small intestine, sānjiāo, bladder, these five are created by sky qi, and their qi reflects sky, therefore they release and do not store* and are known as (chuán huà zhī fǔ) 傳化之府 'the transformational Fu-organs.'" Qi Bo also explains that (pò mén) 魄門 "Gate of Po," a euphemism for the anus, is utilized by the five Zang to expel the turbid.

Definitions: Zang versus Fu

Five Zang	Store jīng-essence and qi, and do not release	Full, not solid
Six Fu	Transport and transform substance, and do not store	Solid, not full

"This is why, when we eat, the stomach becomes solid but the guts are empty. Then when food goes down to be digested, the guts are solid but the stomach is empty."†

Radial pulse, nostril breathing, and patient consent

The Emperor asks, "Why is (qì kǒu) 氣口 'the radial pulse' alone governed by the five Zang?"

Qi Bo answers:

胃者水穀之海, 六府之大源也
(wèi zhě shuǐ gǔ zhī hǎi, liù fǔ zhī dà yuán yě)
Stomach is the sea of grain, the great source of the 6 Fu.

五味入口
(wǔ wèi rù kǒu)
The 5 flavors enter through the mouth,

---

* The 6 Fu receive turbid qi from the 5 Zang.

† 虛 (xū): empty. This is the same character (xū) 虛 as in deficiency from 8 principles diagnosis.

藏於胃以養五藏氣

(cáng yú wèi yǐ yǎng wǔ zàng qì)

[to be] stored in stomach to nourish the five Zangs' qi.

氣口亦太陰也

(qì kǒu yì tài yīn yě)

The radial pulse is also Taiyin.

是以五藏六府之氣味, 皆出於胃

(shì yǐ wǔ zàng liù fǔ zhī qì wèi, jiē chū yú wèi)

Therefore the qi and flavor of five Zang and six Fu all come from stomach.

變見於氣口

(biàn jiàn yú qì kǒu)

Changes are seen at the radial pulse.*

故五氣入鼻

(gù wǔ qì rù bí)

Therefore the five qi enters the nose

藏於心肺

(cáng yú xīn fèi)

[to be] stored in heart and lung.

心肺有病而鼻為之不利也

(xīn fèi yǒu bìng ér bí wéi zhī bú lì yě)

When the heart and lung are diseased, the nose is not clear.

…

---

* 氣口 (qì kǒu): "Qi Mouth." Today clinically we feel the radial pulse at (cùn kǒu) 寸口 for (qì kǒu) 氣口 changes. I am not sure if there is a difference in location or technique between the two.

拘於鬼神者, 不可與言至德

(jū yú guǐ shén zhě, bù kě yǔ yán zhì dé)

Do not speak of virtues to the superstitious.*

惡於鍼石者, 不可與言至巧

(wù yú zhēn shí zhě, bù kě yǔ yán zhì qiǎo)

Do not speak of technique to those averse to acupuncture.†

病不許治者病必不治

(bìng bù xǔ zhì zhě bìng bì bú zhì)

Do not treat those who have not consented to treatment.

治之無功矣

(zhì zhī wú gōng yǐ)

[You will] treat without success.

地勢使然也。

(dì shì shǐ rán yě)

Because of their geography.

---

* 拘於鬼神者 (jū yú guǐ shén zhě): Literally "those limited by ghosts and spirits". According to Henry McCann, who teaches medical classics on both the East and West Coast and practices in New Jersey, this line is significant because the book is clearly departing from the shamanistic origins of Chinese medicine, denying that possession by ghosts or spirits is a legitimate etiology for disease. "Virtues" here can also be translated as "powers" and is the same character (dé) 德 as in the Dào Dé Jīng 《道德經》 Tao Te Jing by Lâo Zǐ 老子.

† Includes needles (acupuncture) and stones (biǎn stone pricking implements, precursors to lancets).

Chapter 12

Discussion on Different Methods and Appropriate Approaches

異法方宜論

(yì fǎ fāng yí lùn)

Chapter 12, Discussion on Different Methods and Appropriate Approaches, is about the healing methods favored by different geographic regions. This chapter reads like a narrative poem.

The Emperor asks, "When doctors treat disease, why do they use different approaches for the same disease?"

Qi Bo replies:

地勢使然也。

(dì shì shǐ rán yě)

Because of their geography.

East
land of fish and salt, coastal water
where sky and earth engender life
the people eat fish and prefer salty
fish make heat in the center
salt consumes blood
therefore folk are dark complexioned
with conditions of *Carbuncles* and *Sores**
best treated by bloodletting stones†

West
land of gold and jade, sand and stone
where sky and land withdraw and collect
the people live on precipices with much wind
robust, tough, needing few clothes
for their rich foods make them fat
therefore exterior pathogens cannot harm their bodies
and their conditions arise from within
best treated by toxic herbs‡

North
where sky and earth are closed and hidden
the land is high, wind is icy
the people enjoy wild places and dairy
making Zang organs *Cold* and conditions of *Fullness*§
best treated by moxibustion¶

---

*　癰 (yōng): carbuncles versus 瘍 (yáng): ulcers.

†　砭石 (biǎn shí): bloodletting stones, often translated as biǎn stones. These are techniques lost, as far as I know.

‡　毒藥 (dú yào): toxic herbs. The character for poison, (dú) 毒 means "toxic but medicinal" here.

§　滿 (mǎn): fullness.

¶　灸炳 (jiǔ bǐng): moxibustion.

South
where sky and land grow and nourish and yang is abundant
the land is low, collecting fog and dew
the people prefer sour and eat fermented foods
therefore they are delicate and red of complexion
prone to *Cramps* and *Impediment**
best treated by fine needles†

Central
where land is flat and damp
where sky and land engender ten thousand crowds
the people eat variously and do not labor
therefore they are prone to *Atrophy, Reversal, Cold, Heat‡*
best treated by exercise§ and bodywork¶

The sage treats using a combination of modalities
as appropriate, curing diseases with different ways.

Contemporary clinical application of Chapter 12

Of course, Qi Bo is referring to regional characteristics of ancient China, but I believe this chapter covers key clinical concepts on which modalities are best for what lifestyle type. We have...

---

* 攣 (luán): *Cramps* versus 痹 (bì): *Impediment.*

† 微鍼 (wēi zhēn): acupuncture. Literally "fine needles," the type of gentle needling with retention most commonly thought of as acupuncture today.

‡ I am not sure if these four characters are two conditions—(wěi jué) 痿厥 *Atrophy Reversal*, i.e. dysfunctional cold limbs, and (hán rè) 寒熱 *Cold Heat*, i.e. alternating chills and fever—or four separate conditions. Based on the northerners whose conditions are all a single character, I am guessing four separate conditions: 痿 (wěi): *Atrophy,* 厥 (jué): *Reversal,* 寒 (hán): *Cold,* 熱 (rè): *Heat.*

§ 導引 (dǎo yǐn): "guided exercise," includes moving meditation, qìgōng, tàijíquán—I suspect that yoga also fits into this definition.

¶ 按蹻 (àn qiào): "bodywork," includes massage and tūiná, probably. Literally "pressing the Qiào" 蹻 as in the Yin/Yang Qiao Vessels of the 8 Extraordinary Vessels.

Modern patients who	Like ancient Chinese
Eat a lot of salt and seafood, maybe even live on a houseboat	Easterners
Are well nourished and physically robust but suffer from internal issues	Westerners
Do not wear enough clothes in ice-cold air conditioned spaces and/or enjoy consuming dairy products	Northerners
Live in basement apartments and/or eat a lot of pickles and sausages	Southerners
Have musculoskeletal issues from being too sedentary	Central Folk

Discussion on Shifting Essence and Changing Qi

移精變氣論

(yí jīng biàn qì lùn)

Chapter 13, Discussion on Shifting Essence and Changing Qi, is about why shamanic healing was sufficient for the ancients but not enough for "current" times (as in, 2000 years ago when the *Huángdì Nèijīng* was being compiled. The Chinese have a tendency to hark back toward a more enlightened Golden Age— even more so than the Greeks).

The Emperor and Qi Bo speak of healing modalities and how, as humanity become less aligned with nature, more elaborate medical interventions become necessary.

Tips on diagnosis

High ancient times*	[People] understood 5 elements, 4 seasons, 8 winds, 6 gatherings. Complexion reflects the sun; pulse reflects the moon. Aligned with (shén míng) 神明 "spirit brightness," therefore death far and life near
Middle ancient times†	8 winds and 5 impediments were treated with 10 days of [herbal] decoctions. If not completely cured, twigs and roots (i.e. plant ends) were used to subdue pathogens with understanding of root and branch
"Contemporary" era‡	Treatments [are given] without understanding of 4 seasons, sun/moon, following/counterflow. Needles are used for exterior, decoctions for interior, therefore new conditions arise before [one is] fully cured

I cannot tell if the rest of this chapter is important, so here is a literal translation of the rest of the conversation, for the reader to decide:

帝曰: 願聞要道
(dì yuē: yuàn wén yào dào)
Emperor says: [I am] willing to hear [of] the Key Way.§

歧伯曰: 治之要極, 無失色脈
(qí bó yuē: zhì zhī yào jí, wú shī sè mài)
Qi Bo says: The utmost key to treatment is not to lose complexion and pulse.

用之不惑, 治之大則
(yòng zhī bú huò, zhì zhī dà zé)
Use/function without confusion, [that is] the great principle to treatment.

---

* 上古 (shàng gǔ) "high ancient times," like the title of *Sùwèn* Chapter 1.

† 中古 (zhōng gǔ) "middle ancient times."

‡ 暮世 (mù shì) "contemporary era," literally "twilight era."

§ 要道 (yào dào): literally, "essential way." 要 (yào) as in 金匱要略 (Jīn Guì Yào Luè) and 道 (dào) as in Daoism.

逆從倒行
(nì cóng dào xíng)
[If you] reverse the movement of counterflow and following,

標本不得
(biāo běn bù dé)
without a grasp of root and branch,

亡神失國
(wáng shén shī guó)
gods will perish and the kingdom will be lost.

去故就新
(qù gù jiù xīn)
Let go of the past and accept the new

乃得真人
(nǎi dé zhēn rén)
To acquire [the wisdom? rank? of a] True Person.

帝曰: 余聞其要於夫子矣
(dì yuē: yú wén qí yào yú fū zǐ yǐ)
Emperor: I hear you speak of the Key.

夫子言不離色脈, 此余之所知也
(fū zǐ yán bù lí sè mài, cǐ yú zhī suǒ zhī yě)
You say not to depart from complexion and pulse, this I know.

歧伯曰: 治之極於一
(qí bó yuē: zhì zhī jí yú yī)
Qi Bo: The utmost treatment is/of one.

帝曰: 何謂一
(dì yuē: hé wèi yī)
Emperor: What [do you mean by] one?

歧伯曰: 一者, 因得之
(qí bó yuē: yī zhě, yīn dé zhī)
Qi Bo: One is gotten by reason.

帝曰: 奈何
(dì yuē: nài hé)
Emperor: Meaning what?

歧伯曰: 閉戶塞牖, 繫之病者
(qí bó yuē: bì hù sāi yǒu, xì zhī bìng zhě)
Qi Bo: Shutter windows [to] connect to the patient

數問其情, 以從其意
(shù wèn qí qíng, yǐ cóng qí yì)
Ask the history several times [to] get the intention/meaning.

得神者昌, 失神者亡
(dé shén zhě chāng, shī shén zhě wáng)
Have spirit, will prosper. Lose spirit, will perish.

帝曰: 善
(dì yuē: shàn)
Emperor: Ah.

The Emperor seems to understand what Qi Bo is talking about here, but I do not.

Discussion on Decoctions and Wines

湯液醪醴論

(tāng yè láo lǐ lùn)

Chapter 14, Discussion on Decoctions and Wines, though ostensibly about water decoctions and medicinal wines, continues the previous dialogue on the sages of time immemorial versus we mortals of contemporary times. The chapter title leads one to expect formulas or recipes for medicinal infusions, but the discussion is actually all theory, quite philosophical.

The Emperor asks about making (tāng yè) 湯液 "water decoctions" and (láo lǐ) 醪醴 "alcoholic infusions" with five grains.

Qi Bo replies, "[You] must use rice grains, and burn rice chaff. Rice grains are complete. Rice chaff is hard."

The Emperor asks why and Qi Bo gives an explanation about rice as the perfect grain because its growth perfectly reflects the appropriate actions of each season: plant in spring, grow in summer, harvest in autumn, store in winter. Because of this, rice symbolizes harmony and balance in seasonal change. The

Emperor then asks why the sages of time immemorial made decoctions and wines but did not use them.

Qi Bo says they made it in preparation but did not need to take it. In the Middle Ancient Times, because virtues were slightly eroded, external pathogens had seasonal advantages, so it was beneficial to take in [the medicine] preventatively.

The Emperor asks, why not in current times?

Qi Bo says, "In current times, [you] must coordinate herbs to attack the center, needles/stone/moxa to treat the exterior."

The Emperor then asks about poor efficacy in the body and Qi Bo answers, "The shén-spirit is not engaged."

Thankfully, this is also confusing to the Emperor, who asks, "What does that mean, the shén-spirit is not engaged?"

Qi Bo explains that if the jīng-essence, shén-spirit, zhì-willpower, and yì-intention are not in alignment with the needles and stone, the condition cannot be cured. He gives an example: "Now jīng-essence is bad and shén-spirit leaves, the nutritive-yíng and defensive-wèi cannot be recovered. Why? Endless addictions and unceasing worries, unsustainable for the spirit, coagulate the nutritive-yíng and expel the defensive-wèi, therefore the shén-spirit leaves, and the disease will not be cured."

The Emperor gives his own example scenario, asking about counterflow* that cannot be treated by acupuncture or herbs.

Qi Bo says, "The disease is the root; the doctor is the branch. If [you] do not have branch and root, the pathogens will not submit."

The Emperor gives another example, not of an exterior invasion but of the exhaustion of the yang of five Zang, leaving corporeal-pò alone with jīng-essence inside, the qi exhausted without and inaccessible within.

Qi Bo recommends balance, moving old blood, warm clothes, using a bloodletting needle "to recover the body," inducing

---

* 逆 (nì): "counterflow." I do not think it is being used as a disease name here. The Emperor defines it as "disease has formed."

sweating and urination* to align the jīng-essence with the season so as to create jīng-essence, to make the bones and flesh preserve the body's own abundance.

---

*   Entertaining euphemism! (kāi guǐ mén) 開鬼門: "opening the ghost doors" means to induce sweating through the pores. (jié jìng fǔ) 潔淨府: "Cleansing the clean house" means to induce urination through the bladder.

Chapter 15

Essentials on the Jade Tablet

玉版論要

(yù bǎn lùn yào)

Chapter 15, Essentials on the Jade Tablet, is about 2 lost texts, *Kuí Duó* 《揆度》 <u>Formulas and Pulses</u>, and *Qí Héng* 《奇恒》 <u>Extraordinary Prognoses</u>. According to Qi Bo, the former is about the depth of illness and the latter is about extraordinary conditions. They are inscribed on a jade tablet, hence the title of the chapter, and are known together as *Hé Yù Jī* 《合玉機》 <u>Convergence of Jade Mechanisms</u>.

Two-part books of classical Chinese medicine

Book title	Part 1 Title	Part 2 Title
Hé Yù Jī 《合玉機》 Convergence of Jade Mechanisms	*Kuí Duó* 《揆度》 Formulas and Pulses	*Qí Héng* 《奇恆》 Extraordinary Prognoses
Huángdì Neijīng 《黃帝 內經》 Yellow Emperor's Internal Classic	*Sùwèn* 《素問》 Plain Questions	*Língshū* 《靈樞》 Magic Pivots
Shānghán Zábìng Lùn 《傷寒雜病論》 Discussion of Cold Damage and Miscellaneous Conditions	*Shānghán Lùn* 《傷寒論》 Discussion on Cold Damage	*Jīn Guì Yào Lüè* 《金匱要略》 Essentials of the Golden Cabinet

Face and pulse reading essentials from Chapter 15

What follows is what appears to be a summary of face and pulse reading essentials from these books:

容色見上下左右, 各在其要
(róng sè jiàn shàng xià zuǒ yòu, gè zài qí yào)
Look at the complexion above, below, right, and left.

其色見淺者, 湯液主治, 十日已
(qí sè jiàn qiǎn zhě, tāng yè zhǔ zhì, shí rì yǐ)
If the color is superficial, it can be treated in 10 days by decoction.

其見深者, 必齊主治, 二十一日已
(qí jiàn shēn zhě, bì qí zhǔ zhì, èr shí yī rì yǐ)
If [the color] is deep, it must be treated in tandem* for 21 days.

其見大深者, 醪酒主治, 百日已
(qí jiàn dà shēn zhě, láo jiǔ zhǔ zhì, bǎi rì yǐ)
If [you] see big deep [colors?], treat with medicinal wine for 100 days.

---

*   By acupuncture and herbs together.

色夭面脫, 不治, 百日盡已

(sè yāo miàn tuō, bú zhì, bǎi rì jìn yǐ)

If the facial complexion is deserted, it is not treatable, and will end in 100 days.

脈短氣絕死

(mài duǎn qì jué sǐ)

Short pulse without qi dies.

病溫虛甚死

(bìng wēn xū shèn sǐ)

Disease warm with extreme deficiency dies.

上為逆, 下為從

(shàng wéi nì, xià wéi cóng)

Up is counterflow, down is following.

女子右為逆, 左為從

(nǚ zǐ yòu wéi nì, zuǒ wèi cóng)

For women, right is counterflow, left is following.

男子左為逆, 右為從

(nán zǐ zuǒ wéi nì, yòu wéi cóng)

For men, left is counterflow, right is following.

易重陽死

(yì chóng yáng sǐ)

Easy [to] double yang, die.

重陰死

(chóng yīn sǐ)

Double yin, die.

Diseases mentioned in Chapter 15

Name	Pulse	Etiology
Impediment Lameness 痹躄 (bì bì)	Broad	Cold and heat mingling
Wasting Qi 消氣 (xiāo qì)	Lone[53]	N/A
Stolen Blood 奪血 (duó xiě)	Deficient leaky	N/A

The method to run *Qí Héng* begins with Taiyin. Running against the control cycle (see Appendix A) is called (nì) 逆 "counterflow." Counterflow causes death. Running with the control cycle (see Appendix A) is called (cóng) 從 "following." Following the flow preserves life.

Discussion on the Essentials of Diagnosis and the End of Channels

診要經終論

(zhěn yào jīng zhōng lùn)

Chapter 16, Discussion on the Essentials of Diagnosis and the End of Channels, answers 2 brief questions posed by the Emperor.

Essentials of diagnosis

The Emperor asks, "What of the essentials of diagnosis?"

Qi Bo answers with calendar correspondences, seasonal needling recommendations, precautions, and consequences, and five Zang needling precautions and consequences. He concludes with a few more tips on needling technique.

Calendar correspondences with qi of sky, land, and human

Months (lunar)	Qi of sky	Qi of land	Qi of human
1–2	Begins to square	Begin to express	At liver
3–4	Proper square	Set to express	At spleen
5–6	Abundant	High	At the head
7–8	Yin qi begins to kill	N/A	At lung
9–10	Yin qi begins to freeze	Begins to close	At heart
11–12	Ice recovers	Closes	At kidney

Seasonal needling recommendations

In spring	Needle (sàn shū) 散俞 Scattered Points[54] and (fēn lǐ) 分理 Muscle Interstices[55]	Stop when blood exits
In summer	Needle (luò shū) 絡俞 Network Points[56]	Stop when see blood
In autumn	Needle the skin along the interstices	Stop when shén-spirit changes
In winter	Needle (shū qiào) 俞竅 Deep Points of (fēn lǐ) 分理 Muscle Interstices	

Seasonal needling precautions and consequences

Mistakes	Consequences
Needle summer in spring	Disrupts the pulse, qi faint, pathogenic factors[57] enters bones and marrow, causing anorexia and shortness of breath
Needle autumn in spring	Sinews cramp, counterflow qi ring, causing cough, periodic shock, and weeping
Needle winter in spring	Pathogens hide, causing distension, and desire to speak
Needle spring in summer	Causes looseness and laziness
Needle autumn in summer	Causes desire in the heart for no words, fear as if about to be arrested

Needle winter in summer	Causes shortness of breath, periodic anger
Needle spring in autumn	Causes forgetfulness of what [one] suddenly gets up to do
Needle summer in autumn	Causes sleepiness and bad dreams
Needle winter in autumn	Causes periodic shivers
Needle spring in winter	Causes sleepiness with insomnia, and visions in sleep
Needle summer in winter	Qi rises, expresses as impediment
Needle autumn in winter	Causes thirst

Five Zang needling precautions and consequences

When needling the chest and abdomen, [we] must avoid the five Zang.

Hit the	Die
Heart	in 1 day
Spleen	in 5 days
Kidney	in 7 days
Lung	in 5 days
Diaphragm	no more than 1 year*

* Causes harm to the center. Even if [treated], patient will die in less than one year.

More tips on the way of needling

- For needling chest and abdomen, use cloth wraps to ensure shallow insertion. If no cure is obtained, needle repeatedly.

- Pricking with needle one must be solemn.

- Shake the needle [to open a hole for pus to come out] when needling a swelling.

- Do not shake [the needle] when needling channels.

The Emperor's second question is phrased more politely, "[I am] willing to hear of the end of 12 channel vessels, may we?"

12 channel vessel death presentations

Vessel of	End*
Taiyang	Eyes roll, opisthotonus, convulsions, color white, sweat, then die
Shaoyang	Ears deaf, all joints slack, eyes staring at outer canthus, complexion first green, then white, then die within 1.5 days
Yangming	Mouth and eyes move, tendency for shock and raving, color yellow, numb, upper and lower channels abundant, then die
Shaoyin	Face black, teeth long and dusty, abdomen distended and shut, no passage upper or lower (unable to eat/defecate?), then die
Taiyin	Abdomen distended shut, no respite, tendency to hiccup and vomit, which then makes counterflow, which then makes the face red. If no counterflow, then no passage upper or lower face black, skin dry, then die
Jueyin	Center hot, throat dry, tendency for incontinence, vexation, in extreme cases, tongue and testicles roll up, then die

---

* 終 (zhōng) "end" versus 絕 (jué) "termination" versus 死 (sǐ) "death."

Discussion on Pulse Essentials and Essence Subtleties

脈要精微論

(mài yào jīng wēi lùn)

Chapter 17, Discussion on Pulse Essentials and Essence Subtleties, is a very detailed account of pulses, which also includes other diagnostics, including complexion (facial diagnosis) and dream interpretations.

Recommended time of day for pulse reading

We begin with Qi Bo's recommendation of reading pulses "at dawn, [when] yin qi has yet to move, yang qi has yet to disperse, food and drink have yet to be consumed, channels and vessels have yet to become abundant, the luò-collateral vessels are harmonious, qi and blood are not chaotic" and progress to pulse indications, complexion indications, and dream interpretation.

Pulse indications

Pulse	Indicates
Long	Qi healed
Short	Qi diseased
Rapid	Heart vexed
Large	Disease advancing
Abundant above	Qi high
Abundant below	Qi distended
Knotted	Qi frail
Thin	Qi scant
Choppy	Heart pain

Complexion indications

Color	Desirable	Undesirable
Red	White wrapping cinnabar	Hematite
White	Goose down	Salt
Green	Old jade	Indigo
Yellow	Gauze wrapping realgar	Sallow earth
Black	Heavy lacquer	Greenish-black*

Diseases mentioned in Chapter 17

Disease	Symptoms
Dampness of Middle Qi 中氣之濕 (zhōng qì zhī shī)	Voice like speaking from inside a room
Stolen Qi 奪氣 (duó qì)	Repeats self when speaking
Shen Disturbance 神明之亂 (shén míng zhī luàn)	Un(der)dressed, speaks inappropriately without boundaries

---

* 地蒼 (dì cāng): I think this is a greenish-black color. **Acu Trivia!** (dì cāng) 地蒼 is the name of acupoint St4.

Doors/Windows Not Holding 門戶不要 (mén hù bú yào)	Cannot retain food
Bladder Not Storing 膀胱不藏 (páng guāng bù cáng)	Cannot stop urinating

	Mansion of	**Symptom**	**Indicates**
Head	Essence and Clarity	Head tilt with vision difficulties	Essence and Spirit [about to be] robbed
Back	Heart and Center	Back bent, shoulders stooped	Fu about to break
Lumbar	Kidney	Cannot turn or shake	Kidney about to expire
Knee	Sinews	Cannot flex or extend knee, compromised gait	Sinews about to expire
Bone	Marrow	Cannot stand for long, also unstable while walking	Bone about to expire

Dream interpretations: excess

Excess	**Dreams of**
Yin	Wading through big water with fear
Yang	Big fire burning
Yin and yang	Mutual killing destruction and harm
Above	Flying
Below	Falling
Full [food]	Giving
Hunger	Taking
Liver qi	Anger
Lung qi	Weeping
Short worms	Gathering crowds
Long worms	Mutual attack ruin and injury

Diagnosis by body part

Seasonal pulse depths

Season	Pulse	Like ~
春 (chūn) Spring	Floats	Fish swimming in ripples
夏 (xià) Summer	At skin	There is surplus everywhere
秋 (qiū) Autumn	Below skin	Hibernating insects about to leave
冬 (dōng) Winter	At bone	Hibernating insects densely packed[58]

More pulses and diseases from Chapter 17

Pulse	Hard and long indicates	Soft and dispersed indicates
Heart	*Aphasia* 舌卷不能言 (shé juǎn bù néng yán)	*Wasting Loop* 消環 (xiāo huán)[59]
Lung	*Hemoptysis* 唾血 (tuò xiě)	*Pouring Sweat* 灌汗 (guàn hàn)
Liver[60]	*Fall as if Struck* 墜若搏 (zhuì ruò bó)	*Overflow Rheum* 溢飲 (yì yǐn)[61]
Stomach[62]	*Fractured Femur* 折髀 (zhé bì)	*Food Impediment* 食痹 (shí bì)
Spleen[63]	*Scant Qi* 少氣 (shǎo qì)	*Leg/Calf Edema* 足胻腫 (zú héng zhǒng)
Kidney	*Fractured Lumbar* 折腰 (zhé yāo)	*Scant Blood*, i.e. anemia 少血 (shǎo xiě)

The Emperor asks about a Heart pulse that is rushing; Qi Bo informs him that it is *Heart Hernia* 心疝 (xīn shàn). They also discuss the Stomach pulse: solid/excess indicates (zhàng) 脹 *Distension*, empty/deficient indicates (xiè) 泄 *Diarrhea*. Then the Emperor asks about disease formation and changes. Qi Bo answers, "Wind becomes (hán rè) 寒熱 *Cold Heat*. (dān) 癉 *Drought* becomes (xiāo zhōng) 消中 *Wasting Center*. (jué) 厥 *Reversal* becomes (diān jí) 巔疾 *Vertex Disease*. (jiǔ fēng) 久風 *Chronic Wind* becomes (sūn xiè) 飧泄 *Lienteric Diarrhea*. (mài fēng) 脈風 *Vessel Wind* becomes (lì) 癘 *Pestilence*. The changes of disease are countless."

The Emperor asks, "Do all (yōng zhǒng) 癰腫 *Carbuncle Swelling*, (jīn luán) 筋攣 *Sinew Cramps*, (gǔ tòng) 骨痛 *Bone Pain* come from this?"

Qi Bo says, "This is swelling from (hán qì) 寒氣 *Cold Qi*, changes from [the] 8 winds."

The Emperor asks, "How to treat?"

Qi Bo says, "These are seasonal conditions; treat with that which controls them to cure."

Chronic versus acute: pulse, complexion

The Emperor asks, "There are old diseases expressed from the five Zang that harm the pulse and complexion, how do we know chronic from acute?"

Qi Bo says, "Excellent question!"

Pulse small complexion same	New disease
Pulse same complexion taken	Chronic disease
Both pulse and complexion taken	Chronic disease
Both pulse and complexion same	New disease

"[If] Liver and Kidney pulse arrive together, complexion [is] green or red, should expect disease of ruin and harm without seeing blood. Visible blood [indicates] damp as if attacked by water."

Diagnostic positions

Qi Bo then describes many diagnostic positions that I do not fully understand. According to Henry McCann, the *Lingshu* has an entire chapter on diagnosing by examining the forearm skin.

Both sides of chǐ	Hypochondria
Outside chi	Kidney
Inside chi	Abdomen center

Left above Fu, outside	Liver
Left above Fu, inside	Diaphragm
Right above Fu, outside	Stomach
Right above Fu, inside	Spleen
Above Fu right, outside	Lung
Above Fu right, inside	Chest center
Above Fu left, outside	Heart
Above Fu left, inside	膻中 (dàn zhōng) Sternum Center*
Before	Anterior
Behind	Posterior
Up above up	Chest and throat
Down below down	Hypogastrium, low back, gluteals, knees, calves, and feet

Pulse images for diseases mentioned in Chapter 17

Condition	Pulse image
Heat Stroke 熱中 (rè zhòng)	Insufficient yin, excess yang
Reversal, Vertex Disease 厥 (jué), 巔疾 (diān jí)	Comes rushed goes slow, solid above empty below
Aversion to Wind 惡風 (wù fēng)	Comes slow goes rushed, empty above solid below
Shaoyin Reversal 少陰厥 (shào yīn jué)	All pulses deep thin rapid
Cold Heat 寒熱 (hán rè)	Deep thin rapid and dispersed
Syncope with Dizziness 眴仆 (xún pū)	Floating and dispersed
Heat 熱 (rè)	All floating but not restless
[Located] at Hand	All floating and restless
[Located] at Yin	All thin and deep, creates bone pain

---

* **Acu Trivia!** (dàn zhōng) 膻中 is the name of acupuncture point R17.

[Located] at Foot	Have quiet
[Located] at Yang vessel	Rapid, moves with one irregularity
Yang qi excess	Excess with choppy, body hot no sweat
Yin qi excess	Excess with slippery, body cold lots of sweating
Yin and yang excess	No sweat, body cold
Heart/Abdominal Accumulation 心腹積 (xīn fù jī)	Push outward but stays in
Body Hot 身熱 (shēn rè)	Push inward but stays out
Low Back/Feet Cool 腰足清 (yāo zú qīng)	Pushes up but does not descend
Head/Nape Pain 頭項痛 (tóu xiàng tòng)	Pushes down but does not ascend
Low Back/Spine Pain 腰脊痛 (yāo jǐ tòng)[64]	Push to bone, scant pulse qi

Discussion on the Balanced Person's Qi and Appearance

平人氣象論

(píng rén qì xiàng lùn)

Chapter 18, Discussion on the Balanced Person's Qi and Appearance, appears to be on breath and pulse. The first paragraph gives us an overview.

The Emperor asks, "How about the balanced person?"

Qi Bo answers with a lecture that takes up the rest of the chapter.

Scant Qi 少氣 (shǎo qi)	1 pulse move with inhalation, 1 pulse move with exhalation
Disease [that is] Warm 病溫 (bìng wēn)	3 pulse moves with inhalation, 3 pulse moves with exhalation, agitated, chi hot
Disease [of] Wind 病風 (bìng fēng)	Same, but chi not hot, pulse slippery
Impediment 痹 (bì)	Same, but pulse choppy
Death 死 (sǐ)	4 pulse moves with exhalation, or pulse not arriving, or suddenly slow and suddenly fast

平人之常氣稟於胃

(píng rén zhī cháng qì bǐng yú wèi)

The balanced person's common/regular qi comes from the stomach.

胃者, 平人之常氣也

(wèi zhě, píng rén zhī cháng qì yě)

Stomach [pulse] is the common qi of the balanced person.

人无胃氣曰逆

(rén wú wèi qì yuē nì)

No stomach qi is called *Counterflow*.

逆者死

(nì zhě sǐ)

Counterflow indicates death.

Spring	Summer	Longsummer	Autumn	Winter	Means
Stomach slightly wiry	Stomach slightly hooked	Stomach faint soft weak	Slightly feathery	Slightly stony	Even
More wiry stomach scant	More hooked stomach scant	More weak stomach scant	More feathery stomach scant	More stony stomach scant	[Zang] disease[65]
Wiry without stomach	Hooked without stomach	Knotted without stomach	Feathery without stomach	Stony without stomach	Death
Stomach but feathery/ autumn	N/A	N/A	Feathery and wiry/ spring	Stony and hooked/ summer	[Other] disease
Stomach but stony	Stomach but stony	Soft weak and stony	N/A	N/A	Winter disease
Extremely stony	Extremely stony	Extremely weak	Extremely wiry	Extremely hooked	Current disease

The (dà luò) 大絡 "great connector" of Stomach is called (xū lǐ) 虛里,* [which] through diaphragm networks lung, exits beneath the left breast and moves the shirt, and is the pulse of (zōng qì) 宗氣 "Ancestral Qi." Abundant, rushed, rapid, interrupted panting indicates (bìng zhōng) 病中 *Disease in Middle*; knotted and horizontal indicates (jī) 積 *Accumulation*; ending without arrival indicates death.

---

* 虛里 (xū lǐ): literally "Empty Mile," located in the fifth intercostal space at the apical pulsation, lateral to St18. I did not know stomach had a great luò; I only knew about spleen's great luò-connecting point, Sp21.

Radial pulse	Disease
Short	*Headache* 頭痛 (tóu tòng)
Long	*Leg/Shin Pain* 足脛痛 (zú jìng tòng)
Rushed upward striking	*Shoulder/Upper Back Pain* 肩背痛 (jiān bèi tòng)
Deep and hard	*Disease in Middle*
Floating and abundant	*Disease in Exterior*
Deep and weak	*Cold Heat, Hernia Conglomeration, Lower Abdominal Pain* 寒熱 (hán rè), 疝瘕 (shàn jiǎ), 少腹痛 (shào fù tòng)
Slippery	*Wind* 風 (fēng)
Choppy	*Impediment* 痺 (bì)
Slow and slippery	*Heat Stroke* 熱中 (rè zhòng)
Abundant and tight	*Distension* 脹 (zhàng)

If pulse follows yin and yang, prognosis is good. If pulse counters yin and yang, prognosis is bad. [When] pulse is aligned with seasons, no other disease [is present. If] pulse is maligned against four seasons, difficult.

Disease	Symptoms
Desertion of Blood 脫血 (tuō xiě)	Many blue-green varicose veins on arm, abundant pulse while lying supine
Lassitude 解㑊 (xiè yì)	Chi pulse slow and choppy
Profuse Sweat 多汗 (duō hàn)	Chi choppy pulse slippery
Diarrhea 後泄 (hòu xiè)	Chi cold pulse thin
Heat Stroke 熱中 (rè zhòng)	Chi rough and frequently hot

Zang	Time
Liver	庚辛 (gēng xīn)
Heart	壬癸 (rén guǐ)
Spleen	甲乙 (jiǎ yǐ)
Lung	丙丁 (bǐng dīng)
Kidney	戊己 (wù jǐ)

True Zang manifestations that lead to death

"Pulses counter to the season [are] difficult to treat."

Season	Pulse
Spring/Summer	Skinny
Autumn/Winter	Floating big
Disease	**Pulse**
Wind Heat	Quiet
Diarrhea/Bloodloss	Solid
Disease at Middle	Deficient
Disease at Exterior	Choppy hard

Definition of pulse with no stomach qi: liver not wiry, kidney not stone-like.

Discussion on True Zang of the Jade Mechanisms

玉機真藏論

(yù jī zhēn zàng lùn)

Chapter 19, Discussion on True Zang of the Jade Mechanisms, expands on the pulse diagnostics in Chapter 18, with a detailed description of each of the four seasonal pulses and corresponding symptoms of excess and deficiency. The Emperor asks about each one, ending with the central earth pulse of spleen. I have omitted literal translations here because I lack deep insights into pulse reading. Also, I believe that the radial pulse readings we do today hail more from the Classic of Difficulties, though the textures described in the Nànjīng are similar to the ones described in Chapter 7: spring is wiry, summer is hooked, autumn is feathery, winter is something deep called (yíng) 營. This is a good passage to study if you want descriptions of pulse textures.

Then the Emperor stands suddenly and makes obeisance to his physician Qi Bo in gratitude for the important essentials of pulse reading, stating that he will inscribe the changes of pulse and 5 complexions, *Kuí Duó* 《揆度》 <u>Formulas and Pulses</u> and *Qí Héng* 《奇恆》 <u>Extraordinary Prognoses</u>, the 2 lost books from Chapter 15 which are 2 parts of the book called *Hé Yùjī* 《合玉機》 <u>Convergence of Jade Mechanisms</u>, on the jade tablet (which he also mentioned in Chapter 15) with the intent to reread daily.

Each Zang receives qi from that which it generates (i.e. child), and passes [qi] to that which is controlled by it (i.e. grandchild); the qi lives in that which it generates (i.e. mother) and dies of that which it does not control (i.e. grandparent).

Generation and controlling cycles of the five Zang
Liver receives qi from heart, passes to spleen, qi lives in kidney, arrives at lung then dies
Heart receives qi from spleen, passes to lung, qi lives in liver, arrives at kidney then dies
Spleen receives qi from lung, passes to kidney, qi lives in heart, arrives at liver then dies
Lung receives qi from kidney, passes to liver, qi lives in spleen, arrives at heart then dies
Kidney receives qi from liver, passes to heart, qi lives in lung, arrives at spleen then dies

This is how death by counterflow occurs. Divide 1 day and 1 night into 5 parts.

The oft quoted "Wind is the elder of a hundred diseases"* is here in this chapter, at the beginning of a passage on the etiology of wind-generated conditions in the body, including (fēi bì) 肺痹 *Lung Impediment*, (gān bì) 肝痹 *Liver Impediment* AKA 厥 (jué) *Reversal*, (pí fēng) 脾風 *Spleen Wind* AKA 癉 (dān) *Drought*, (shàn jiǎ) 疝瘕 *Hernia Conglomerations* with (shào fù yuān rè) 少腹冤熱 *Hypogastric Veiling Heat* and pain with white exudate AKA 蠱 (gǔ) *Possession*, and 瘛 (chì) *Clonic Convulsion*, i.e. grand mal seizure.

There is a long passage on the true Zang pulse presentations and the various deaths that ensue. The Emperor reiterates which seasonal pulses are aligned with the season, and which are

---

* 「風者, 百病之長也。」 (fēng zhě, bǎi bìng zhī zhǎng yě) "Wind is the elder of a hundred diseases."

considered counterflow to the season. Finally, Qi Bo explains the five excess deaths [signs] (pulse abundant, skin hot, abdomen distended, no excretion or urination, visual distortions) versus five deficient deaths [signs] (pulse thin, skin cold, qi scant, diarrhea and incontinence, inability to eat or drink). If consuming porridge stops the diarrhea/incontinence, the deficient patient lives. If sweating induces bowel movements, then the excess patient lives.

Discussion on the Three Parts and Nine Indicators

三部九候論

(sān bù jiǔ hòu lùn)

Chapter 20, Discussion on the Three Parts and Nine Indicators, though also about pulses, is named after pulse positions beyond the radial pulse commonly used in pulse diagnosis today. Reading the radial pulse at Lu9 was not common practice until the *Nàn Jīng* 《難經》 Classic of Difficulties was written in the late Han Dynasty, sometime after the *Nèijīng* but before the *ShānghánLùn*.

The Emperor asks a long question about the nine needles. Qi Bo compliments the question and answers, "This is the ultimate numerology between heaven and earth."*

---

* 歧伯對曰:「妙乎哉問也!此天地之至數。」 (qí bó duì yuē: miào hū zāi wèn yě! cǐ tiān dì zhī zhì shù)

The Emperor replies, "[I am] willing to hear of the ultimate astrology between heaven and earth, how it converges in the human body, and how the throughput of blood and qi informs prognosis."*

So Qi Bo counts for him, "The ultimate numerology between heaven and earth begins with 1 and ends with 9. 1 is sky, 2 is land, 3 is human, and each have 3 parts; 3 times 3 is 9, to reflect 9 wilds.† Therefore humans have 3 parts, each part has 3 indicators, to decide death and life, to take care of a hundred diseases."

Of course, the Emperor immediately asks, "What are the 3 parts?"

Qi Bo answers, "Lower, middle, upper. Each part has 3 indicators: sky, land, human." He then gives anatomical positions for each, in the following order:

Part	Reflection	Position	Reflects
Upper	Sky	Arterial pulse of bilateral foreheads	Head
Upper	Land	Arterial pulse of bilateral cheeks	Mouth and teeth
Upper	Human	Arterial pulse anterior to ears	Ears and eyes
Middle	Sky	Hand Taiyin	Lung
Middle	Land	Hand Yangming	Chest center
Middle	Human	Hand Shaoyin	Heart
Lower	Sky	Foot Jueyin	Liver
Lower	Land	Foot Shaoyin	Kidney
Lower	Human	Foot Taiyin	Spleen and stomach

---

* 帝曰:「願聞天地之至數。合於人形, 血氣通, 決死生, 為之奈何。」 (dì yuē: yuàn wén tiān dì zhī zhì shù, hé yú rén xíng, xiě qì tōng, jué sǐ shēng, wéi zhī nài hé).

† 九野 (jiǔ yě): "9 wilds", a term in Chinese astrology for the 9 sections of the sky that contains the 28 constellations.

The Emperor then asks about signs determining death and life and Qi Bo lists:

Body abundant pulse thin, not enough qi and short of breath	Danger
Body thin pulse big, too much qi in chest	Die
Body and qi proportionate	Live
Examination [findings] in threes and fives (i.e. mismatched and confused)	Disease
3 parts, 9 indicators all misaligned	Die
Upper, lower, right and left pulses reflect as if ground by pestle	Gravely ill
Upper, lower, right and left pulses not aligned and cannot be counted	Die
Center pulse aligned with itself but not others	Die
Center pulse relatively decreasing	Die
Eyes sunken	Die

The Emperor asks, "How do we know where the disease is located?"

Qi Bo says, "Observe the single small pulse of the 9 indicators, [this indicates] disease.* [One] must first know the pulse of the channel, and then know the pulse of the condition.† When Foot Taiyang qi is exhausted, the legs cannot flex or extend, and death must come with eyes rolled up."

The Emperor asks, "What of winter yin and summer yang?"

Qi Bo answers, "Of the 9 indicators' pulses, all deep, thin, suspended, reversed are yin, corresponding to winter; therefore [patient] dies at midnight. Abundant, restless, panting, rapid are yang, corresponding to summer; therefore [patient] dies at noon. Therefore those with *Cold Heat* disease die at dawn, those

---

*   In fact, single small, large, rushed, late, hot, cold, or sunken pulses all indicate disease. There is more on palpating the lower leg to differentiate disease or not diseased, and reflection misalignments (1 = disease, 2 = dire disease, 3 = terminal disease).

†   I have omitted a sentence here on true Zang pulse and death.

with *Heat Stroke* and *Heat Disease* die at noon, those with *Wind Disease* die at dusk, those with *Water Disease* die at midnight."*

The Emperor then asks about treatment approaches for the treatable cases. Qi Bo answers, "When the meridian is diseased, treat the jīng-channels. When the collaterals are diseased, treat the luò-vessels. When the blood is diseased and the body hurts, treat the channels and collaterals. If the condition is extraordinary, then bloodlet the Extraordinary Vessels. If there is excess above and deficiency below, palpate to find knotted luò-vessels and bleed out the blood. When blood is visible, [the luò collateral] is clear. Pupils high means Taiyang is insufficient. Eyes rolled up means Taiyang is exhausted. You must observe this, for it determines death or life. Finger and 5 fingerwidths up from lateral wrist and retain needle."

There is much of this chapter that I do not comprehend. Was that last sentence a point prescription?

---

*   I have omitted a few sentences here about not dying, i.e. not fatal prognoses.

Addendum on Channels and Vessels

經脈別論

(jīng mài bié lùn)

Chapter 21, Addendum on Channels and Vessels, is about the effects and affects of courage, timidity and food ingested. It includes pulse images for using lower hé-sea points* and the pathophysiology of five kinds of sweat.

The first paragraph discusses courage and timidity as observational diagnosis, and the different types of sweat:

Causes	Sweat
Overeating	Stomach
Shock robs jing-essence	Heart

---

* 下俞 (xià shū): literally "lower acupoints" here refers to 下合穴 (xià hé xuè) the "lower convergent points" that we mistranslate as hé-sea points. I opted for the common mistranslation so as not to confuse readers, but (hé) 合 means "to come together." 合 is a pictograph of hands together over a mouth open in prayer, and has never meant "sea" or "ocean"; that is (hǎi) 海 as in (hǎi zǎo) 海藻.

Carry heavy distant travel	Kidney
Sprinting out of fear	Liver
Physical labor	Spleen

The second paragraph tracks the qi and jīng-essence of food ingested through the body, the first type of sweat mentioned in the paragraph above. The locations read like a flowchart:

Food qi → Stomach → Liver → Sinews
Yin qi → Stomach → Heart → Vessels
Vessel qi channels → Lung → Skin → Fu → 5 Zang → vertebrae → Radial pulse
Beverages → Stomach → Spleen → up to Lung, or down to Bladder

The last paragraph is a summary of what happens when a certain Zang (dú zhì) 獨至 "arrives alone." I think this is a pulse image. I believe this section is giving us tips on when to use the lower hé-sea points.

Zang	Arrives alone, causing
Taiyang	Reversal panting empty qi counterflow Etiology: yin deficient/yang excess Treatment: drain exterior and interior with lower shū
Shaoyang	Reversal of qi before Qiao suddenly big Treatment: drain yang and tonify yin with lower shū
Taiyin	5 vessels qi scant, stomach not even Treatment: tonify yang and drain yin with lower shū
Jueyin	True deficiency with qi reversal and white sweat Treatment: adjust food and herbs, treat with lower shū

Zang	Corresponding [pulse] image
Taiyang	3 yang: floating
Shaoyang	1 yang: slippery but not solid
Yangming	Big floating, Taiyin pulse drum, Kidney deep not floating

Discussion on Zang Qi and Season Laws

藏氣法時論

(zàng qì fǎ shí lùn)

Chapter 22, Discussion on Zang Qi and Season Laws, returns to five elements for nutritional/dietary recommendations.

The first section tells us which flavors to eat for issues in the five Zang.

Zang	Governs	Treated by	Heavenly Stems
Liver	Spring	Foot Jueyin/Shaoyang	甲乙 (jiǎ yǐ)
	If liver is urgent, eat sweet to slow it		
Heart	Summer	Hand Shaoyin/Taiyang	丙丁 (bǐng dīng)
	If heart is slow, eat sour to astringe it		
Spleen	Longsummer	Foot Taiyin/Yangming	戊己 (wù jǐ)
	If spleen is damp, eat bitter to dry it		

Lung	Autumn	Hand Taiyin/ Yangming	庚辛 (gēng xīn)
	If lung qi counterflows, eat bitter to drain it		
Kidney	Winter	Foot Shaoyin/Taiyang	壬癸 (rèn guǐ)
	If kidney is dry, eat spicy to moisten it		

The next section tells the seasonal and daily/hourly prognosis of disease given in the language of the 10 Heavenly Stems located in each of the five Zang. It gives prognoses of what time of day a patient is likely to worsen or improve. It also details which flavors will create what actions on said condition. This is a good section to study for enthusiasts of chronobiology.

Then follows a section on symptoms of each of the five Zangs' diseases.

	Symptoms	If deficient, then	Treatment
Liver	*Hypochondriac Pain* radiating to hypogastrium *Tendency to Anger*	*Poor Vision* *Impaired Hearing* Fearful as if about to be arrested (*Paranoia*)	Choose corresponding channels Jueyin, Shaoyang
~ Qi Counterflow	*Headache* *Deafness* *Cheek Swelling*		Bleed Jueyin, Shaoyang channels
Heart	*Chest/Center Pain* *Costal Fullness* *Hypochondriac Pain* *Upper Back/Scapular Pain* *Inner Arm Pain*	*Chest/Abdominal Enlargement* *Hypochondriac Pain* radiating to lower back	Take corresponding channels Shaoyin/ Taiyang
Blood in sublingual veins means disease is changing			Bleed UB40
Spleen	*Body Heaviness* Tendency for *Muscular Atrophy, Gait Changes, Clonic Convulsions, Foot Sole Pain*	*Abdominal Fullness* *Borborygmus* *Lienteric Diarrhea*	Bleed Taiyang, Yangming, Shaoyin channels

Lung	*Cough, Panting Counterflow Qi Shoulder/Upper Back Pain Sweating Sacrum, Gluteals, Knees, Hips, Thighs, Calves, Feet Pain*	*Shortness of Breath Deafness Esophageal Dryness*	Bleed Taiyin, Foot Taiyang external, Jueyin internal
Kidney	*Abdominal Enlargement* with lower leg swelling *Panting, Cough Body Heaviness Night Sweats Aversion to Wind*	*Chest/Center Pain Abdominal Pain Cold Feet Lack of Joy*	Bleed Shaoyin Taiyang

Finally, the colors from Chapter 4 are reiterated and their recommended foods and flavors are detailed.

Announcing and Clarifying the Five Qi

宣明五氣

(xuān míng wǔ qì)

Chapter 23, Announcing and Clarifying the Five Qi, reads like lists.

Five entries

Sour	Liver
Spicy	Lung
Bitter	Heart
Salty	Kidney
Sweet	Spleen

Symptoms that manifest in the five qi

Heart	噫 (yī) burps
Lung	欬 (ké) coughs
Liver	語 (yǔ) speaks
Spleen	吞 (tūn) swallows
Kidney	欠 (qiàn) yawns and 嚏 (tì) sneezes

Five diseases

Stomach	*Qi Counterflow*, *Reflux*, and *Fear*
Large and small intestine	*Diarrhea*
Lower jiāo	*Overflows to Water* (a disease name that includes edema, I think)
Bladder	Not flowing creates *Retention*, not conserving creates *Incontinence*
Gallbladder	*Tendency to Anger*

Five unions

When jīng-essence qì unites with:	Then
Heart	Joy
Lung	Sorrow
Liver	Worry
Spleen	Timid
Kidney	Fear

Five aversions

Heart	Dislikes heat
Lung	Dislikes cold
Liver	Dislikes wind
Spleen	Dislikes damp
Kidney	Dislikes dry

Five fluids

Heart	Sweat
Lung	Snot
Liver	Tears
Spleen	Drool
Kidney	Spittle

Five flavors' taboos

Flavor	Enters	If it is diseased	Then avoid eating too
Spicy	Qi	Qi	Spicy
Salty	Blood	Blood	Salty
Bitter	Bones	Bones	Bitter
Sweet	Flesh	Flesh	Sweet
Sour	Sinews	Sinews	Sour

Blood, Qi, Body, Emotions

血氣形志

(xiě qì xíng zhì)

Chapter 24, Blood, Qi, Body, Emotions, enumerates the abundance of qi and blood in each channel, (biǎo lǐ) 表裡 exterior-interior pairs, the back-shū point locations, and general recommended treatment modalities. Neither the Emperor nor Qi Bo is mentioned; it is another purely informative chapter.

Blood versus qi proportions in six channels

Taiyang	More blood, less qi
Shaoyang	Less blood, more qi
Yangming	More blood, more qi
Shaoyin	Less blood, more qi
Jueyin	More blood, less qi
Taiyin	Less blood, more qi

Yin-Yang of hand and foot channels

Hand channels		Foot channels	
Taiyang	Shaoyin	Taiyang	Shaoyin
Shaoyang	Jueyin	Shaoyang	Heart Master
Yangming	Taiyin	Yangming	Taiyin

Now [we] know the troubles of hand foot yin yang, to treat [we] must first get rid of the blood to get rid of the trouble, offer what is desired, and then drain the excess and mend* the insufficient.

To measure the back-shū, first measure between the two nipples, fold in the middle, and then divide roughly in half: this is the measure of 2 yǔ, i.e. 25 percent of the distance between the nipples.

Location of back-shū points

1 yǔ above is even with Du-14†	
~ below	shū of ~
2 yǔ‡	Lung
1 dù§	Heart
1 dù	Liver/Spleen¶
1 dù	Kidney

---

* 補 (bǔ): "to mend," often translated as "to tonify."

† **Acu Trivia!** 大椎 (dà zhuī): Chinese name of C7/Du14, literally "big vertebra."

‡ The text actually says "2 yǔ below, level with the under yǔ." I guess we can replace yǔ with vertebral height.

§ 1 (dù) 度 = 2 (yǔ) 隅 below, level with the under yǔ.

¶ Liver on the left, Spleen on the right.

Five body emotions

	Body (xíng) 形	Emotions (zhì) 志	Source of disease	Treatment
1.	Happy	Troubled	Vessels	Moxibustion/ Acupuncture
2.	Happy	Happy	Flesh	Needles/Stone*
3.	Troubled	Happy	Sinews	Compresses/ Stretching†
4.	Troubled	Troubled	Throat	Herbs
5.	If the body has experienced repeated shock and fright, the channels and collaterals are blocked, and disease is generated by numbness, treat with massage and tinctures/liniments			

Six channel treatment qi and blood reasoning

Needle Yangming [when it is safe] to expel blood and qi
Needle Taiyang to expel blood without damaging qi
Needle Taiyin to expel qi without damaging blood
Needle Shaoyin to expel qi without damaging blood
Needle Jueyin to expel blood without damaging qi

---

* 石 (shí) "stone." For bloodletting, a sharpened stone implement.

† 熨引 (yùn yǐn). This is 熨 (yùn) as in hot iron 熨斗 (yùn dǒu) and 引 (yǐn) as in guided 導引 (dǎo yǐn). I know there are tàijí and qìgōng 導引 (dǎo yǐn) practices, so perhaps a better translation would be hot compresses and guided therapeutic exercises.

Discussion on Treasuring Life and Integrating Form

寶命全形論

(bǎo mìng quán xíng lùn)

Chapter 25, Discussion on Treasuring Life and Integrating Form, is about how humans are reflections of heaven and earth. There are lines about the mandate of heaven,* how the 12 (jíé) 節† channels/meridians of humans reflect the yin and yang of the sky, and how our deficiencies and excesses reflect the "cold and heat of the sky" (i.e. the weather).

---

* Throughout this chapter (and many others), "heaven" and "sky" are the same character (tiān) 天.

† 節 (jié): originally a character that meant bamboo node, here (jié) 節 has several possible meanings: channels, musculoskeletal joints, solar terms, but I am not sure which.

Some interesting *verbs* on overacting

伐 (fá)	Wood is *chopped* down by metal
滅 (miè)	Fire is *extinguished* by water
達 (dá)	Earth *arrives/achieves* via wood
缺 (quē)	Metal *wanes* because of fire
絕 (jué)	Water is *terminated* by earth

Priorities of treatment

1. Treat the shén-spirit
2. Nourish the body
3. Know the truth of poisons versus medicine
4. Know the size of biǎn stones
5. Know the blood and qi of Fu and Zang

These five methods each have their advantages.*

The rest of the chapter consists of guidelines on how to treat human conditions in resonance with the natural rhythms of heaven and earth. After listing the five priorities of treatment, Qi Bo mentions that "in contemporary needling, everyone knows to tonify the deficient and drain the full"† and that there are benefits to "moving in resonance with heaven and earth, harmonizing like sounds [echoes?], following like shadows."‡

---

* 「五法俱立, 各有所先。」 (wǔ fǎ jù lì, gè yǒu suǒ xiān)

† 「今末世之刺也, 虛者實之, 滿者寫之, 此皆眾工所共知也。」 (jīn mò shì zhī cì yě, xū zhě shí zhī, mǎn zhě xiè zhī, cǐ jiē zhòng gōng suǒ gòng zhī yě)

‡ 「法天則地, 隨應而動, 和之者若響, 隨之者若影。」 (fǎ tiān zé dì, suí yìng ér dòng, hé zhī zhě ruò xiǎng, suí zhī zhě ruò yǐng)

帝曰: 願聞其道。

(dì yuē: yuàn wén qí dào.)

The Emperor says, "[I] am willing to hear of the Way of this."

歧伯曰: 凡刺之真, 必先治神

(qí bó yuē: fán cì zhī zhēn, bì xiān zhì shén)

Qi Bo says, "The truth of needling [is that one] must first treat the shén-spirit."

He goes on with a very poetic description of acupuncture technique that involves "the ability to play with alternations"* and...something to do with a crossbow bolt,† perhaps waiting for the right moment to intervene?

Chapter 25 ends with one of my favorite quotes, on how to hold a needle:

深淺在志,

(shēn qiǎn zài zhì,)

The depth is in the will.

遠近若一,

(yuǎn jìn ruò yī,)

distance and proximity are as one.

如臨深淵,

(rú lín shēn yuān,)

As if approaching a deep abyss,

手如握虎,

(shǒu rú wò hǔ,)

holding a tiger in hand,

神無營於眾物。

(shén wú yíng yú zhòng wù.)

let the spirit be not encamped among the host of things.

---

* 「可玩往來」 (kě wán wǎng lái): this is the same (wǎng lái) 往來 as in Xiǎo Chái Hú Tāng 小柴胡湯's key symptom "alternating cold and heat" (wǎng lái hán rè) 「往來寒熱」 (Shānghán Lūn: line 96)

† 「伏如橫弩, 起如發機」 (fú rú héng nǔ, qǐ rú fā jī)

Discussion on Eight Proper Spiritual Clarities

八正神明論

(bā zhèng shén míng lùn)

Chapter 26, Discussion on Eight Proper Spiritual Clarities, deals with needling in accordance with the sun, the moon, and the stars.

Weather's effect on blood/wèi qi

(tiān) 天 **Weather**	(rì) 日 Sun	(xiě) 血 **Blood**	(wèi qì) 衛氣 **Defensive qi**
(wēn) 溫 Warm	(míng) 明 Bright	(nào yè) 淖液 Liquid	(fú) 浮 Floats[66]
(hán) 寒 Cold	(yīn) 陰 Cloudy	(níng qì) 凝泣 Coagulates	(chén) 沈 Sinks

The relation of moon phases to the body and treatment taboos

Moon	Body	Do not	Consequences
Waxes	Blood and qi begin to [distill into] jīng-essence, defensive-wèi qi begins to move [67]	Drain	(zàng xū) 藏虛 *Zang Deficiency*
Full	Solid (shí) 實, muscles firm	Tonify	(chóng shí) 重實 *Double Excess*[68]
Wanes	Muscles diminish, channels empty, defensive qi leaves, form alone remains	Treat	(luàn jīng) 亂經 *Disrupted Channels*

There is a passage here about the stars and the eight winds* (i.e. environmental influences of the eight cardinal directions), then a bit more discourse on the difference between superior doctors (shàng gōng) 上工 and inferior doctors (xià gōng) 下工. "The superior doctor knows the temperature of the sun, the phase of the moon, the four seasons' depth of qi, sees that which is invisible to others, and uses the 3 parts and 9 indicators to nip diseases in the bud and save that which has not yet been defeated. When [a patient] exerts the body, (còu lǐ) 腠理 'the interstices' open and becomes susceptible to wind."

Then follows an interesting paragraph about using (fāng) 方 "square" to drain and (yuán) 員 "circle" to tonify. It specifies that fāng and yuán do not indicate needle types. I do not know what square and circle refer to.

Definitions of (xíng) 形 form versus (shén) 神 spirit

形 (xíng): ask about disease, palpate the channel, can be seen, i.e. tangible

神 (shén): inaudible, eyes bright, heart open, willpower leads [to] epiphany that cannot be verbalized, i.e. intuitive. All is murky, then suddenly bright, like wind blowing clouds away

---

* **Acu Trivia!** 八風 (bā fēng): eight winds is the set of eight extra points between the toes.

Separation and Convergence of True and Evil

離合真邪

(lí hé zhēn xié)

Chapter 27, Separation and Convergence of True and Evil, is about exterior invasions and the basics of how to treat them using acupuncture. The first section uses weather as an extended metaphor for the human body. Then follows a description of technique, the earliest historical description in Chinese medical literature of using a needle to manipulate qi without bloodletting.

On needling to disperse AKA (dé qì) 得氣 "getting qi"

吸則內鍼, 無令氣忤
(xī zé nèi zhēn, wú lìng qì wǔ)
Insert needle on inhalation to avoid insulting the qi.

靜以久留, 無令邪布

(jìng yǐ jiǔ liú, wú lìng xié bù)

Retain [the needle] long to prevent pathogen from spreading.

吸則轉鍼, 以得氣為故

(xī zé zhuǎn zhēn, yǐ dé qì wéi gù)

Rotate needle on inhalation until the qi arrives.

候呼引鍼, 呼盡乃去

(hòu hū yǐn zhēn, hū jìn nǎi qù)

Wait for exhalation to guide needle, remove needle at end of exhalation.

大氣皆出, 故命曰寫

(dà qì jiē chū, gù mìng yuē xiè)

Great qi [will] all exit. This is known as draining.

The Emperor asks, "What about tonifying* insufficiency?" Qi Bo answers with a sentence about palpation, applying finger pressure, followed by the instruction that the needle should be inserted at the end of exhalation and removed on inhalation followed by "pushing the door closed to keep shen and qi preserved." He does not mention rotating the needle, and instead of (dé qì) 得氣, he describes waiting for the qi to arrive.†

On needling to tonify AKA (hòu qì) 候氣 "awaiting qi"

呼盡內鍼

(hū jìn nèi zhēn)

Insert the needle at the end of exhalation,

---

* 補 (bǔ): usually translated as "tonify." This is the character for "patching up/mending" or "completing a garment" made of the radical for garment (yī) 衤 next to (fǔ) 甫, a pictograph of a sprouting field which was also the honorific for a great man because it sounds like (fù) 父 "father" (*Shuō Wén Jiě Zì*).

† This is the first mention of needling to manipulate qi without changing the blood.

靜以久留

(jìng yǐ jiǔ liú)

retain quietly for a long time,

以氣至為故

(yǐ qì zhì wéi gù)

wait for the qi to arrive,

如待所貴

(rú dài suǒ guì)

as if waiting for someone highly valued,

不知日暮

(bù zhī rì mù)

not knowing dusk [has fallen].

The Emperor asks about awaiting qi, and Qi Bo explains. The Emperor understands him better than I do, for he says, "Ah," and moves on to another topic, "However, if the waves do not arise, do we await the qi in vain?"

Qi Bo gives some other techniques one can do in the meantime, and cautions that misuse of the draining technique in acupuncture can damage the true qi of a person.

Chapter 28

Discussion on the Complete Evaluation of Deficiency and Excess

通評虛實論

(tōng píng xū shí lùn)

Chapter 28, Discussion on the Complete Evaluation of Deficiency and Excess, defines and expands on deficiency and excess in pulses and how they manifest in patients. First, the Emperor asks for definitions of (xū) 虛 and (shí) 實. Qi Bo answers, "Pathogens abundant is (shí) 實. Essence qi robbed is (xū) 虛."

Next the Emperor asks how (xū) 虛 and (shí) 實 manifest. The answers become more clinical and complex, involving pulses.

Qi Bo says, "Qi deficient [presentation indicates] lung deficiency. Qi counterflow [creates] cold feet. If it is not the season, [patient will] live. If it is the season [(i.e. autumn?), patient will] die."

The Emperor asks, "What about when the channels and collaterals are both (shí) 實 excess? How would [we] treat?"

Qi Bo answers, "When both channels and collaterals are excess, the cùn-inch pulse is urgent and the chǐ-cubit pulse is moderate; treat accordingly. Slippery indicates following, choppy indicates counterflow...if the five Zangs' bones and flesh are slippery and uninhibited, that is sustainable."

The Emperor asks, "If the luò-collateral qi is insufficient, but the jīng-channel qi has surplus, what then?"

Qi Bo answers, "When luò qi is insufficient and jīng qi has surplus, the cùn-inch pulse is hot and the chǐ-cubit pulse is cold. In autumn and winter, this is counterflow, in spring and summer this is following. Treat the main condition."

The Emperor asks, "What if the channel is deficient but the collaterals are full?"

Qi Bo says, "If the channels are deficient and the collaterals are full, the chǐ-cubit pulse will be hot and the cùn-inch pulse will be cold and choppy. Spring and summer die, autumn and winter live...for full collaterals and deficient channels, moxa the yin and prick the yang. For full channels and deficient collaterals, prick the yin and moxa the yang."

The Emperor asks, "What is double deficiency?"

Qi Bo says, "Pulse is deficient in both inch and cubit...if it is slippery, the patient will live. If it is choppy, the patient will die."

Now we move into a section where the Emperor poses many possible presentations and Qi Bo gives prognoses based on what the pulses reveal.

Pulse prognoses

Presentation	Pulse	Prognosis
Cold qi violently rises	Full and solid	Solid and slippery, live. Solid and counterflow, die
Hand/Feet cold, head hot	Solid full	Spring/Autumn live. Winter/Summer die. Pulse floating and choppy with heat in the body, die

Form entirely full	Urgent, big, hard, chǐ choppy and unresponsive	Following (i.e. hands/feet warm), live. Counterflow (i.e. hands/feet cold), die
Infant with *Heat* (rè) 熱 Infant with *Wind-Heat* (fēng rè) 風 熱 and *Panting* (chuǎn) 喘	Suspended small	Hands/Feet warm, live. Hands/ Feet cold, die
	Solid big	Slow [pulse], live. Urgent, die
Intestinal Blockage (cháng pǐ) 腸癖 with hematochezia		Body hot, die. [Body] cold, live
Intestinal Blockage with white foam in stools	Deep	Live
	Floating	Die
Intestinal Blockage with pus and blood in stools	Suspended faint	Die
	Slippery big	Live
Intestinal Blockage without heat in body	Not suspended faint	Slippery big, live. Suspended choppy, die
Vertex Disease (diān jí) 巔疾	Wide big slippery	Will gradually heal on its own
	Small hard urgent	Fatal, cannot be treated
	Deficient	Can be treated
	Excess	Die
Wasting Drought (xiāo dān) 消癉	Solid big	Can be treated
	Suspended small hard	Cannot be treated

The Emperor then poses a question about the (dù) 度 measurement of form, bone, vessel, and sinews and answers himself* with, "In spring, treat the luò-connecting points. In summer, treat the shū-stream points. In autumn, treat the six Fu.† In winter...use herbs and minimize needles/stones." There are some specific exceptions about needling less in the winter,

---

*   Future scholars surmise that we might be missing Qí Bó's answer here.

†   Some commentators, like Zhāng Jièbīn 張介賓, believe (liù fǔ) 六府 "six Fu" means any point on the yang meridians of the six Fu. Others believe it refers to hé-sea points.

mostly for various (yōng) 癰 *Carbuncles*, but also for (huò luàn) 霍亂 *Sudden Chaos* and (xián) 癇 *Seizures*. Unfortunately, instead of point names, the text describes combinations like "needle Hand Taiyin each 5, needle [of?] Taiyang 5, needle Hand Shaoyin jīng luò beside 1, Foot Yangming 1, up ankle 5 cùn needle 3."* I am not sure which acupoints are being referred to here, and there appears to be no consensus among future scholars who annotated the work, so I am omitting the point prescriptions.

Etiology of disease presentations

Disease Presentation	Etiology
消癉 (xiāo dān) *Wasting Drought* 仆擊 (pū jī) *Syncope* 偏枯 (piān kǔ) *Asymmetrical Withering*, aka hemiplegia 痿厥 (wěi jué) *Atrophy Reversal* 氣滿發逆 (qì mǎn fā nì) *Qi Full Expressing Counterflow* 肥貴人 (féi guì rén) *Fat Highborn Person*	Fatty rich diet
隔 (gé) *Continuous Vomiting* 塞 (sāi) *Congestion* 閉 (bì) *Block* 絕 (jué) *Termination* 上下不通 (shàng xià bù tōng) *Inhibition Above and Below*	Sudden violent anxiety
暴厥 (bào jué) *Violent Reversal* with (lóng) 聾 *Deafness* 偏塞 (piān sāi) *Asymmetrical Congestion* 閉不通 (bì bù tōng) *[Urinary] Block and Inhibition*	Internal qi violently thinned
中風 (zhòng fēng) *Wind Strike* not due to internal causes	Lingers because of slenderness
蹠跛 (zhí bǒ) *Sole Limp*	Cold wind damp
黃疸 (huáng dǎn) *Jaundice* 暴痛 (bào tòng) *Acute Pain* 巔疾 (diān jí) *Vertex Disease* 厥 (jué) *Reversal* 狂 (kuáng) *Mania*	Long-standing counterflow Five Zang not balanced Six Fu congested
頭痛 (tóu tòng) *Headache* 耳鳴 (ěr míng) *Tinnitus* 九竅不利 (jiǔ qiào bú lì) *9 Orifices† Inhibition*	Digestive organs

---

* This is the point prescription for (xián jīng) 癇驚 *Seizure Shock*.

† The nine orifices include two eyes, two ears, two nostrils, mouth, anus, and urethral opening.

Discussion on Taiyin Yangming

太陰陽明論

(tài yīn yáng míng lùn)

Chapter 29, Discussion on Taiyin Yangming, explains why the earth organs do not have a specific season, and what the difference is between disease in the spleen versus disease in the stomach. First there are some more tidbits on yin versus yang.

	Yang	Yin
Qi of	Sky	Land
Master of	External	Internal
Path is	Solid	Empty
Receives	Exterior pathogens	Irregular diet/lifestyle
Enters	Six Fu	Five Zang

	Yang	**Yin**
Disease presentation	*Body Hot* (shēn rè) 身熱 *Sleep at Odd Hours* (bù shí wò) 不時臥 *Asthma* (chuǎn hū) 喘呼 in upper [jiāo]	*Bloating* (chēn) 䐜 *Fullness* (mǎn) 滿 *Blockage and Congestion* (bì sè) 閉塞 *Lienteric Diarrhea* (sūn xiè) 飧泄 in lower [jiao] which can become chronic *Intestinal Blockage* (cháng pǐ) 腸癖
~ governs ~	喉 (hóu) Pharynx/Sky Qi	咽 (yān) Larynx/Land qi
Receives	Wind qi	Damp qi
Qi travels	From feet up to head, then down arms to fingertips	Hands up to head, then down to feet
Condition travels	Up and then down*	Down and then up*

*This is why *Wind Damage* presents above initially and *Damp Damage* presents below initially.

The Emperor asks, "Why do the four limbs lose function when spleen is diseased?"

Qi Bo says, "The four limbs receive qi from the stomach... when spleen is diseased and unable to move the fluids for the Stomach, the four limbs do not get grain qi. Therefore, the vessels are inhibited. The sinews, bones and muscles have no qi with which to function."

The Emperor asks, "Why does spleen not have a season?"

Qi Bo explains that spleen is earth and governs the center, and is hidden between each of the four seasons for 18 days each. It is not particular to any one season, but the spleen as a Zang supports the jīng-essence of the stomach, earth. Because all things grow from the earth, therefore [it reaches] from head to foot.

The Emperor asks, "Spleen and stomach are connected by membranes, and therefore can transport fluids, how does this work?"

Qi Bo says, "Foot Taiyin is 3 yin; its vessel goes through the stomach, belongs to spleen, and networks the esophagus,* therefore Taiyin moves the qi for the 3 yin. Yangming is exterior, the sea of five Zang and six Fu, therefore it moves the qi for the 3 yang. All Zang and Fu organs receive qi from the Yangming through their channels, therefore they transport fluids for the stomach." He reiterates how, if the four limbs do not receive grain qi, the vessels become inhibited, the sinews, bones, and muscles have no qi with which to generate, and therefore atrophy into dysfunction.

---

* 嗌 (yì): esophagus.

An Explanation of the Yangming Vessel

陽明脈解

(yáng míng mài jiě)

Chapter 30, An Explanation of the Yangming Vessel, is an adorably short chapter, which I now realize my favorite acupuncture points teacher quoted at us constantly while I was doing my master's program at the Academy of Chinese Culture and Health Sciences in Oakland, California. The chapter is a very vivid word-picture of what happens when the Foot Yangming Stomach is diseased and the patient becomes "averse to people, fire, frightened by sounds of wood (but not the sounds of metal bells or drums)."* When the condition gets dire, the patient may even "rip off clothes [while] walking, climb high and sing, ingest nothing for days, trespass

---

* 「惡人與火, 聞木音則惕然而驚, 鐘鼓不為動」 (wù rén yǔ huǒ, wén mù yīn zé tì rán ér jīng, zhōng gǔ bù wéi dòng)

over walls and atop buildings not usually scalable...rave and curse with no regard for personal boundaries."*

My teacher mostly spoke of this set of symptoms as analogous to (kuáng) 狂 the manic part of (diān kuáng) 癲狂 *Withdrawal/ Mania*, but the *Sùwèn* here ascribes the etiology to stomach.[†] The presentation here described fits all the (chéng qì tāng) 承氣湯 laxative formula options from the <u>Discussion of Cold Damage</u>.

---

*   「棄衣而走, 登高而歌, 或至不食數日, 踰垣上屋, 所上之處, 皆非其素所能... 妄言罵詈, 不避親疎」 (qì yī ér zǒu, dēng gāo ér gē, huò zhì bù shí shù rì, yú yuán shàng wū, suǒ shàng zhī chù, jiē fēi qí sù suǒ néng....wàng yán mà lì, bú bì qīn shū).

†   The description of the Stomach Channel from *Lingshu* Chapter 10 echoes this.

Discussion on Heat

熱論

(rè lùn)

Here is the disease (shāng hán) 傷寒 *Cold Damage* that the
(*Shānghán Lùn*) 《傷寒論》 by Zhāng Zhòngjǐng 張仲景 is
all about! However, Chapter 31 is rather misleadingly titled
Discussion on Heat.

The Emperor begins, "Current conditions of *Heat* are all *Cold
Damage* type, and of recovery and death, death always happens in
6–7 days, recovery in 10+ days. Why is this?"

Qi Bo answers, "Juyang* is where all yang belongs. [Its] vessel
connects to Du16, and therefore masters qi for all yang. When
a person is damaged by cold, the disease is hot." I wonder if the
days are exact, to be taken literally,† or metaphorical, but at first
glance the six channels diagnosis laid out in this chapter appears
to be analogous to the *Shānghán Lùn*. A closer look at the notable
symptoms for each syndrome reveals that only the names are the

---

* 巨陽 (jù yáng): literally "giant yang," an alternative name for Taiyang.

† Henry McCann is of the opinion that the dates are not literal but metaphorical
references to duration.

same; all three yang diseases are exterior and therefore analogous to the *Shānghán Lùn*'s Taiyang Disease.

Symptoms of *Cold Damage*

Cold Damage	Channel	Symptoms
Day 1	Juyang	Head and Nape pain, low back and spine stiff
Day 2	Yangming	Body hot, eyes ache, nose dry, cannot sleep
Day 3	Shaoyang	Chest and ribs hurt, ears deaf
Day 4	Taiyin	Abdomen full and throat dry
Day 5	Shaoyin	Mouth and tongue dry, thirsty
Day 6	Jueyin	Vexation, fullness, and retracted testicles
Day 7	Juyang improves	Headache slightly better
Day 8	Yangming improves	Body heat slightly better
Day 9	Shaoyang improves	Hearing slightly better
Day 10	Taiyin improves	Belly deflates as before and appetite returns
Day 11	Shaoyin improves	Thirst stops, no fullness, tongue dry, sneezing
Day 12	Jueyin improves	Testicles relieved, lower abdomen descends slightly

The Emperor then asks about patients who present with (yí) 遺 *Loss** and Qi Bo explains that this is actually a sign of recovery too, caused by forcibly eating when the heat was still extreme.

---

* 遺 (yí) *Loss*: involuntary discharge of...urine? Feces? Sperm? Leukorrhea? I am not sure which.

Pulse and presentation of
"Two [channels?] affected by *Cold*"

Day 1	Juyang + Shaoyin	Headache, mouth dry, vexation fullness
Day 2	Yangming + Taiyin	Abdominal fullness, body heat, no appetite, raving
Day 3	Shaoyang + Jueyin	Ears deaf, testicles withdrawn, reversal, cannot eat or drink, cannot recognize people, die in 6 days

Cold Damage transforms to *Warm Diseases*

The Emperor asks, "When the five Zang are damaged, the six Fu are not clear, the nutritive and defensive are not circulating, and [the patient] dies in 3 days, why is this?"*

Qi Bo says, "Yangming is the eldest of the 12 channels, with abundant blood and qi, therefore [the patient] does not recognize people. In 3 days, the qi is exhausted, therefore [the patient] dies. For cases of *Cold Damage* that turns warm: before summer solstice this is known as (wēn bìng) 溫病 *Warm Disease*; after summer solstice this is known as (shǔ bìng) 暑病 *Summerheat Disease*. Summerheat will release itself with sweating, do not try to stop it."†

---

* 「五藏已傷，六府不通，榮衛不行，如是之後，三日乃死，何也。」(wǔ zàng yǐ shāng, liù fǔ bù tōng, róng wèi bù xíng, rú shì zhī hòu, sān rì nǎi sǐ, hé yě).

† 「陽明者，十二經脈之長也，其血氣盛，故不知人，三日其氣乃盡，故死矣。凡病傷寒而成溫者，先夏至日者為病溫，後夏至日者為病暑，暑當與汗皆出，勿止。」(yáng míng zhě, shí èr jīng mài zhī zhǎng yě, qí xiě qì shèng, gù bù zhī rén, sān rì qí qì nǎi jìn, gù sǐ yǐ. fán bìng shāng hán ér chéng wēn zhě, xiān xià zhì rì zhě wéi bìng wēn, hòu xià zhì rì zhě wéi bìng shǔ, shǔ dāng yǔ hàn jiē chū, wù zhǐ).

Pricking Heat

刺熱

(cì rè)

Chapter 32, Pricking* Heat, is actually not so much about acupoint prescriptions as diagnosis again, especially facial diagnosis, how to treat before *Heat* has arisen.

Signs and symptoms for *Heat Disease* in each Zang, with channel prescriptions

	Presentation	Heat conflicts† then	Needle
Liver	Urine yellow, abdominal pain, more sleep, body hot	Manic speech and shock, hypochondriac pain, restless limbs, inability to sleep soundly	Foot Jueyin Shaoyang
Heart	No joy, then after a few days heat [presents]	Sudden heart pain, vexation, chest oppression, retching, headache, face red, no sweat	Hand Shaoyin Taiyang

---

*   I chose to translate (cì) 刺 as "pricking" rather than "needling" because to needle should be (zhēn) 針.

†   爭 (zhēng) "conflicts, at odds with."

Spleen	Head heavy, cheeks hurt, emotions vexatious, complexion green, wants to retch, body hot	Low back pain with inability to function, flex or extend, abdominal fullness, diarrhea, bilateral jowl pain	Foot Taiyin Yangming
Lung	Shivers and reversal, hairs stand on end, averse to wind and cold, tongue coating yellow, body hot	Pant and cough, pain in chest, breast, and upper back, shallow breathing, extreme headache, sweat followed by chills	Hand Taiyin Yangming: bleed size of soybean for immediate relief
Kidney	Low back pain, calves sore, bitter thirst, copious drinking, body hot	Nape painful and stiff, calves cold and sore, soles of feet hot, taciturnity	Foot Shaoyin Taiyang

For all sweating, needle that which overacts on it to induce sweating.

Facial diagnosis for *Heat Disease*

Zang	Liver	Heart	Spleen	Lung	Kidney
~ turns red first	Left cheek	Face	Nose	Right cheek	Jowls

If you see the color change and needle before the disease expresses, this is known as treating before disease has arisen. In lighter cases, the complexion may not change. With proper treatment [the patient] may recover within 3 weeks. Repeated wrong treatments result in death.

To treat *Heat Disease*, first have [the patient] drink cold water, then needle. Have them wear cooler clothing and stay in a cold place until the body cools down.

Channel prescriptions for other presentations

Presentation	Needle
Chest and hypochondriac pain, restless limbs	Foot Shaoyang, Tonify Foot Taiyin, in extreme cases 59 pricks
Hand/Arm pain	Hand Yangming Taiyin until sweating, then stop
Begins at foot/calf	Foot Yangming until sweating, then stop
Body heavy, bone pain, deafness, blurry vision	Foot Shaoyin, in extreme cases 59 pricks

Dizzy and then feverish, chest and hypochondriac fullness	Foot Shaoyin Shaoyang

Pulse diagnosis/prognosis for *Heat Disease*

Presentation	Diagnosis/Prognosis
Taiyang Pulse Complexion manifest on cheekbones	*Heat Disease*
Not yet manifest, get sweaty	Waiting for the correct time to heal
Seen in conflict with Jueyin Pulse	Die within 3 days
Shaoyang Pulse Complexion manifest in front of cheeks	*Heat Disease* with Kidney involvement
Not yet manifest, get sweat	Waiting for correct time to heal
Seen in conflict with Shaoyin Pulse	Die within 3 days

Back point prescriptions for *Heat*

Acupoint[69]	Treats Heat in
Beneath third thoracic vertebra (Du12/UB42)	Chest center
Beneath fourth thoracic vertebra (Du11.5/UB43)	Diaphragm
Beneath fifth thoracic vertebra (Du11/UB44)	Liver
Beneath sixth thoracic vertebra (Du10/UB45)	Spleen
Beneath seventh thoracic vertebra (Du9/UB46)	Kidney

Facial diagnosis for other conditions in Chapter 32

Complexion	Diagnosis
Counterflow beneath cheeks (up to cheekbone)	*Big Conglomeration* 大瘕 (dà jiǎ)
Lower teeth	*Abdominal Fullness* 腹滿 (fù mǎn)
Behind cheekbones	*Hypochondriac Pain* 脇痛 (xié tòng)
Above cheeks	[Disease located] *Above Diaphragm* 膈上 (gé shàng)

Discussion on Evaluating Heat Disease

評熱病論

(píng rè bìng lùn)

I am not sure how to translate this chapter title, but it is something like Discussion on Judging/Critiquing/Evaluating Heat Disease. In actuality, the Emperor and Qi Bo appear to be analyzing in more detail some specific cases, so maybe the title would be better translated as Case Studies of Heat Disease or Further Comments on Heat Disease. This is why I do not want to commit to a single translation. How can we begin to understand the shape of things if we flatten their complexity into something we can readily comprehend?

In Chapter 33, Discussion on Evaluating Heat Disease, the Emperor describes the presentation of four specific *Heat Diseases* and Qi Bo explains each condition and the etiology of observable signs and symptoms, as well as treatment.

(yīn yáng jiāo) 陰陽交 *Yin-Yang Exchange*

Presentation: (bìng wēn) 病溫 *Warm Disease*, after induced sweating heat (fever?) returns, pulse restless and/or racing and does not weaken after sweating, manic speech, inability to eat

Etiology: sweating comes of food; food comes of jīng-essence. When external pathogens exchange conflict between bones and flesh to create sweating, this indicates that jīng-essence is victorious over the pathogens. If jīng-essence is victorious, [the patient] should be able to eat and heat should not return
Heat = pathogens
Sweat = jīng-essence
Recurrent Heat = pathogens winning
Unable to eat = no resources for jīng-essence
This is why Discussion on Heat says, "After sweating, if the pulse is still restless and exuberant, death." When pulse does not match sweating, the disease is winning, and death follows
Manic speech = losing coherence.[70] Those who lose coherence also die

Treatment: we see 3 deaths and not 1 life, therefore patient must die, even if we cure the disease

(fēng jué) 風厥 *Wind Reversal*

Presentation: body hot, sweaty, vexed and full. (fán mǎn) 煩滿 *Vexation Fullness* is not relieved by sweating

Etiology:
Sweating but body still hot = (fēng) 風 *Wind*
Sweating and still vexed/full = (jué) 厥 *Reversal*
Juyang governs qi, therefore it receives pathogens first
Shaoyin is its biǎo-lǐ pair, and goes up when heated, causing *Reversal*

Treatment: needle biǎo-lǐ and drink decoction

(láo fēng) 勞風 *Taxation Wind*

Presentation: stiff above, vision blurred, spittle like snot, averse to wind, shudders

Treatment: flex and extend 3–7 days. Cough out thick pellet of greenish-yellow snot either from the mouth or nose, otherwise [the phlegm] damages lung, resulting in death

(shèn fēng) 腎風 *Kidney Wind*

Presentation: facial edema, damaged speech

Treatment: if deficient, do not needle, otherwise creates 風水 (fēng shuǐ) *Wind Water* within 5 days

(fēng shuǐ) 風水 *Wind Water*

Presentation: shortness of breath, periodic heat from chest/upper back to head*, sweating, hands hot, mouth dry, bitter thirst, urine yellow, eyes puffy below, abdominal borborygmus, body heavy, difficult to walk, amenorrhea, vexation, inability to eat, cannot sleep supine without coughing fits

Etiology:
shortness of breath, hot flashes and sweating = Yin deficiency
Urine yellow = Heat in lower abdomen
Cannot lie supine = Stomach disharmony
Coughing when supine = [qi] ascends to (pò) 迫[71] "press" the lung
Puffiness below eyes = (shuǐ qì) 水氣 *Water Qi*, because water is yin, and the area beneath the eyes is also yin. If there is water in the abdomen, the area beneath the eyes must be puffy
True qi counterflows upward = mouth bitter tongue dry, cannot lie supine without coughing up clear water. All diseases of water [share the symptom of] inability to sleep, if sleep then shock and coughing fits ensue
Borborygmus = disease root at stomach
Vexed, unable to eat = thin spleen, separation between stomach and abdominal cavities
Body heavy, difficulty walking = Stomach vessels at feet
Amenorrhea = (bāo mài bì) 胞脈閉 Uterus Vessel Blocked[†]

---

*　hot flashes!

†　The Uterus Vessel belongs to Heart and connects to the center of the uterus. When qi ascends to (pò) 迫 "press" Lung, Heart qi cannot descend through, therefore the period does not come.

Discussion on Regulating Counterflow

逆調論

(nì tiáo lùn)

Chapter 34, Discussion on Regulating Counterflow, is a similar format as Chapter 33. The Emperor asks questions about certain symptoms or clinical presentations and Qi Bo answers. The first section addresses abnormal body temperatures; the second section is about insomnia and shortness of breath (snoring?) both in the sense of (xī yǒu yīn) 息有音 "breathing audibly" and (chuǎn) 喘 "panting," which I usually think of as asthma.

Disease presentation and etiology mentioned in Chapter 34

Presentation	Disease	Etiology
Body unusually warm or hot	*Heat* 熱 (rè) plus *Vexation Fullness* 煩滿 (fán mǎn)	Yin qi < yang qi
Body cold as if just coming out of water despite warm clothes, without external pathogenic symptoms	*Impediment Qi* 痹氣 (bì qì)	Yang qi < yin qi
Limbs hot as if on fire with *Wind Cold*, muscles waste	N/A	Yin qi deficient, Yang qi excess
Body cold, soup and fire cannot heat, thick clothes cannot warm, but patient does not shiver, joints cramp	*Bone Impediment* 骨痹 (gǔ bì)	Kidney water < liver/heart fire; *Cold goes into bones*[72]
Flesh numb, even if wearing clothes (i.e. warm enough), still flesh feels numb	*Death*[91] 死 (sǐ)	Nutritive qi deficient, Defensive qi excess[92]

Presentation	Etiology
Cannot sleep, breathing audible	Yangming (stomach) counterflow upward[93]
Cannot sleep but breathing quiet	Sea of 6 Fu (stomach) qi not descending[93]
No insomnia, breathing audible	Lung collaterals counterflow
Cannot sleep, short of breath when supine	Water qi guesting

Discussion on Ague

瘧論

(nuè lùn)

Chapter 35, Discussion on Ague, begins with the etiology and presentation of *Ague* in terms of cold and heat, yin and yang. Nigel Wiseman, the author of <u>A Practical Dictionary of Chinese Medicine</u>, and a UK-born translator living in Taiwan who specializes in Chinese medical terminology, translates (nuè) 瘧 as *Malaria* but I think that nuè is not limited to what we call malaria in biomedicine; it can be any condition marked by intermittent fevers, such as PMS, Mono, or Lyme Disease. Likewise, the old Chinese (dān) 癉, often translated to *Diabetes* which I call *Drought*, is not exactly equivalent to Type 2 Diabetes Mellitus (T2DM), though many cases of (xiāo dān) 消癉 *Wasting Drought*, marked by increased hunger and thirst, resemble Type 2 Diabetes Mellitus. However, that is a whole other book.

Pathogenesis and presentation of (nuè) 瘧 *Ague*

Pathogenesis	Presentation
Yangming deficient	Cold shivers
Juyang deficient	Low back, upper back, head, nape pain
3 yangs deficient	Bone pain, internal cold
Yang exuberant	External heat
Yin deficient	Internal heat
Both external/internal heat	Panting and thirst with desire to drink cold beverages

Qi Bo explains that all ague arises from summerheat injury during summer, when the nutritive qi runs closer to the surface and the interstices are open. At the transition to autumn, open pores + wind + bathing leads to (shuǐ qì) 水氣 "water qi" residing in the skin alongside defensive qi, traveling the yang by day, yin by night.

The Emperor then asks about episodes that cycle every other day (i.e. (jiē nuè) 痎瘧 *Intermittent Ague*) and Qi Bo explains that this is because the yin is caught inside conflicting with yang, and only the yang expresses.

The Emperor asks about the difference between episodes at sunset versus sunrise. Qi Bo says if the pathogens are lodged at Du16 then it expresses at sunset; if they are lodged in the spine or the Zang, the condition expresses at different times. Then there is a passage on defensive qi and opening the interstices to treat pathogens residing in the head and nape that gives us context for (fēng) 風 *Wind* versus (nuè) 瘧 *Ague*. *Wind* is always present; *Ague* is intermittent.

(hán nuè) 寒瘧 *Cold Ague*

Etiology: *Cold Damage* followed by *Wind Damage*

Presentation: first chills, then fever

(wēn nuè) 溫瘧 *Warm Ague*

Etiology: *Wind Damage* followed by *Cold Damage*

Presentation: first fever, then chills

Pathogenesis: *Wind Strike* in winter, cold qi hides between bone and marrow, in spring when yang qi expresses, the pathogen cannot escape, [then] great summerheat leads to brain/marrow/muscle wasting, interstices drain. Alternately, overexertion leads to pathogens/sweat exiting simultaneously. This condition hides in the Kidney; its qi travels outward from inside

(dān nuè) 癉瘧 *Drought Ague*

Etiology: yin qi ends first, yang qi expresses alone

Presentation: shortness of breath, vexation, hands and feet hot, retching

Pathogenesis: constitutional lung heat + *Reversal* counterflowing upward, interstices open due to exertion, *Wind Cold* lodges in the skin and muscle layers, expressing with exuberant qi (only heat signs, no cold). The qi hides in heart and causes wasting, which is why it is called *Drought Ague*

Although *Ague* is usually contracted at the end of summer or beginning of autumn, it can also occur against the seasons, and will present as follows.

Seasonal onset of *Ague*

Contracted in	Autumn	Winter	Spring	Summer
Presentation	Extreme cold	Not very cold	Averse to wind	Profuse sweating

Chapter 36

Pricking Ague

刺瘧

(cì nuè)

Like Chapter 33, Chapter 36, Pricking Ague, is a very practical guideline on when it is appropriate to needle which channels for various types of *Ague*. There is a lot of bloodletting in the recommended treatments.

Ague treatment protocols: six channels

Ague of	Symptoms	Needle
Foot Taiyang	Low back pain, head heavy, cold on back followed by heat, then sweat nonstop	UB40[94]
Foot Shaoyang	Body lassitude neither too cold nor too hot, dislikes people, fearful	Foot Shaoyang[95]
Foot Yangming	First cold for long time, then hot, likes sunlight, moonlight and fire	St42
Foot Taiyin	Unhappy, frequent sighs, no appetite, more cold, if hot then sweat[96]	N/A

Ague of	Symptoms	Needle
Foot Shaoyin	Vomit a lot, extreme cold heat, heat > cold, want to close windows and doors and stay in, difficult prognosis	N/A
Foot Jueyin	Low back pain, hypogastrium full, urine retentive, frequent bowel movements	Foot Jueyin[97]

Ague treatment protocols: Five Zang and Stomach

Organ	Signs and Symptoms	Treatment
Lung	Heart cold, cold [when] extreme [transforms to] heat, tendency for shock, as if hallucinating	Hand Taiyin Yangming
Heart	Vexatious, desire [for] cool water, cold > heat	Hand Shaoyin
Liver	Complexion greenish blue, sighs, as if dead	Bleed Foot Jueyin
Spleen	Cold, abdominal pain, heat causes borborygmus, then sweat	Foot Taiyin
Kidney	Shivery, lumbar spinal pain with difficult defecation, eyes dizzy, cold hands and feet	Foot Taiyang/Shaoyin
Stomach	Hungry but cannot eat, or bloated	Foot Yangming/Taiyin varicosities

Ague treatment protocols: other signs and symptoms

There are a few more passages about needling options, mostly involving bloodletting technique.

Ague with	Treatment
Body just starting to express heat	Bleed UB42
Body just starting to express cold	Needle Hand/Foot Yangming Taiyin
Pulse full and big	Bleed back-shū
Pulse small and solid	Moxa calf Shaoyin, needle finger jǐng-well
Pulse slow, big, empty	Herbs, no acupuncture
Pulse disappears	Bleed between fingers[98]
Not cured within 3 treatments	Bleed sublingual veins[99]
Not cured after bloodletting sublinguals	Bleed UB40 and [Huà Tuó] Jiá Jǐ

Ague treatment protocols based on onset

In treating 瘧 (nuè), it is important to ask about the onset and treat appropriately.

Onset	Treatment
Headache/Head heavy	Needle top of head (Du20?), two [on the] forehead (GB14? St8?), two between eyebrows (UB2)
Nape/Upper back pain	Needle [content lost]
Low back/Spine pain	Bleed UB40
Hand/Arm pain	Needle Hand Shaoyin Yangming and between fingers
Foot/Calf pain	Needle Foot Yangming and between
Sweating with aversion to cold[100]	Needle three yang channels back-shū
Shin sore and tender to palpation	Bleed GB38 with (chán zhēn) 鑱鍼 "chisel needle"
Body slightly painful	Needle UB67

Ague treatment protocols with unusual symptoms

Ague with	Treatment
All yin jǐng-wells do not bleed	Needle every other day
No thirst, expresses every other day	Needle Foot Taiyang
Thirsty, expresses every other day	Needle Foot Shaoyang
(wēn nuè) 溫瘧 *Warm Ague* without sweat	59 Pricks

I do wonder if Lyme can be called (nuè) 瘧 *Ague*. Henry McCann agrees that the symptoms are sufficiently similar.

Discussion on Qi Reversal

氣厥論

(qì jué lùn)

Chapter 37, Discussion on Qi Reversal, covers the effects of pathogenic Cold or Heat moving from one Zang to another and all their disease names.

Mutual movements of Cold and Heat in the Five Zang and Six Fu

~ moves Cold	To	Disease
Kidney	Liver	*Carbuncle Swelling* 癰腫 (yōng zhǒng) *Scant Qi* 少氣 (shǎo qì)
Spleen	Liver	*Carbuncle Swelling* 癰腫 (yōng zhǒng) *Sinews Cramp* 筋攣 (jīn luán)

Liver	Heart	*Mania* 狂 (kuáng) *Blocked Middle* 隔中 (gé zhōng)
Heart	Lung	*Lung Wasting* 肺消 (fèi xiāo)[101]
Lung	Kidney	*Bubbling Water* 湧水 (yǒng shuǐ)[102]
Spleen	Liver	*Shock Nosebleed* 驚衄 (jīng nù)
Liver	Heart	*Death* 死 (sǐ)
Heart	Lung	*Diaphragm Wasting* 膈消 (gé xiāo)
Lung	Kidney	*Soft Tetany* 柔痙 (róu jìng)
Kidney	Spleen	*Deficiency* 虛 (xū) *Intestinal Blockage* 腸澼 (cháng pì)[103]
Uterus	Bladder	*Dribbling* 癃 (lóng) *Hematuria* 溺血 (niào xiě)
Bladder	SI	*Oral Putrefaction* 口糜 (kǒu mí)[104]
SI	LI	*Anxiety Conglomeration* 慮瘕 (lǜ jiǎ) *Sinking* 沈 (chén)
LI	Stomach	*Food Changes* 食亦 (shí yì)[105]
Stomach	GB	also *Food Changes* 食亦 (shí yì)
GB	Brain	*Burning Ethmoid* 辛頞 (xīn è) *Nasal Discharge* 鼻淵 (bí yuān)[106]

Discussion on Coughs

欬論

(ké lùn)

Chapter 38, Discussion on Coughs, is one of the first chapters I read on my own. It is very straightforward.

黃帝問曰: 肺之令人欬, 何也。

(huáng dì wèn yuē: fèi zhī lìng rén ké, hé yě.)

The Emperor asks, "Why does the Lung make people cough?"

歧伯對曰: 五藏六府, 皆令人欬,

(qí bó duì yuē: wǔ zàng liù fǔ, jiē lìng rén ké,)

Qi Bo answers, "The 5 Zang and 6 Fu [can] all make people cough,

非獨肺也。

(fēi dú fèi yě.)

not just the Lung."

Qi Bo then explains all the differentials of cough symptoms for the Zang and Fu organs.

Cough of 5 Zang

Onset	First affects	Symptoms	In extreme cases
Autumn	Lung	Cough with wheezing sound	Spit blood
Summer	Heart	Cough with Heart pain, choking sensation in throat	Sore throat/swelling
Spring	Liver	Cough with bilateral rib pain	Cannot laterally rotate[107]
Ultimate Yin	Spleen	Cough with right rib pain that refers to the shoulders and [mid] back	Cannot move, moving causes extreme coughing fits
Winter	Kidney	Cough with low back and mid-back pain	Cough up saliva

If 5 Zang coughs become chronic, they move to the corresponding Fu.

Cough of 6 Fu

Zang	Moves to	Symptoms	In extreme cases
Spleen	Stomach	Cough with retching	Cough up longworms
Liver	Gallbladder	Cough/Retch up bile	N/A
Lung	LI	Fecal incontinence when coughing	N/A
Heart	SI	Pass gas when coughing	N/A
Kidney	Bladder	Urine incontinence when coughing	N/A
Chronic	Sānjiāo	Cough with abdominal fullness, lack of appetite or thirst[108]	N/A

Treating cough

For Zang, treat the shū-stream:* for Fu, treat the hé-sea; for swelling, treat the jīng-river.

---

* 俞 (shū) here may be back-shū or shū-stream (usually (shū) 輸); those two characters were sometimes used interchangeably back when the Sùwèn was written. I believe it is shū-stream because of the other point suggestions

Chapter 39

Discussion on Lifting Pain

舉痛論

(jǔ tòng lùn)

Chapter 39, Discussion on Lifting Pain, describes various patterns of pain: sudden pain, pain that is better with pressure, pain that is not better with pressure, and so on. Almost all of the examples have to do with cold except the last one, which has to do with heat. It also gives us an overview of visual diagnosis/ palpation for pain, and how emotions affect qi movement.

The first paragraph uses the super polite question and answer format that we have not seen since early chapters. The Emperor begins with some insights that do not appear at first glance to have anything to do with medicine. "I have heard that those who enjoy speaking of the sky (i.e. meteorologists) must have verification with humanity; those who enjoy speaking of the past (i.e. historians)* must have context in the present; those who enjoy speaking of people (i.e. gossips) must dislike something

---

* Wáng Bīng believes this refers to ancient sages who knew how to nourish life.

about themselves.* Now I ask you, in order [for one] to speak of the comprehensible, see the visible, palpate the tangible, in order [for one] verify through personal experience and thereby relieve confusion. [I am] willing to hear the Way of this."

Qi Bo makes formal obeisance and answers, "Of what (dào) 道 [do you] ask?"

The Emperor says, "[I] wish to hear of (cù tòng) 卒痛 *Sudden Pain* in the 5 Zang, and which qi causes each." Qi Bo answers that *Sudden Pain* is caused by cold qi lodged in channels, which causes delays (i.e. stagnation). Outside the vessels, this creates (shǎo xiě) 少血 *Scant Blood*. Inside the vessels, this creates (qì bù tōng) 氣不通 *Qi Stagnation*.

Pathogenesis of pain

Pain	Pathogenesis
Suddenly ceases	Cold qi guests outside vessels, leading to capillaries contracting[109]
Extreme, unceasing	Heavy/Repeated *Cold Strike* (zhòng hán) 中寒 †
Extreme, tender to palpation	Cold qi guests in channels and vessels,[110] creating vessel fullness
Stops with palpation	Cold qi guests between Intestines and Stomach, below abdominal membrane, trapping blood in capillaries[111]
Palpation does not benefit	Cold qi guests in vessels along spine, pressing cannot reach
Palpable throbbing	Cold qi guests in Penetrating Vessel,[112] leads to vessel congestion
Radiates to Heart and upper back	Cold qi guests in vessels of back-shū, leads to poor circulation, leads to [local] blood deficiency. Also, the back-shū pours into Heart[113]

---

*   There is one sentence here about (dào) 道 "the Way" that I do not comprehend.

†   This could also be read as (zhōng hán) 中寒 center cold, i.e., middle jiao [deficient] cold; I'm not sure which translation is better. Maybe they both apply.

Radiates to hypochondria and lower abdomen	Cold qi guests in vessels of Jueyin, which wrap around the genitals and link to Liver, leading to poor circulation and contracted veins

Pain	Pathogenesis
Abdominal, radiates to genitals and buttocks	Cold qi guests in genitals and buttocks, rises to lower abdomen, and leads to poor circulation
Chronic, leads to *Accumulation*	Cold qi guests in SI membranes and inside blood of capillaries, leads to poor circulation, blood cannot enter channels
Sudden, with syncope	Cold qi guests in 5 Zang, *Reversal* counterflows upward draining leads to yin qi exhausted, yang qi not yet entered[114]
With retching	Cold qi guests in Stomach and Intestines, *Reversal* counterflow exits upward
Abdominal with diarrhea	Cold guests in SI, leads to SI unable to gather [stools]
With urine retention	Heat guests in SI, leads to *Drought*, *Heat*, thirst, and dries [urine]

We see a new character, (jiǒng) 炅 that is a (rì) 日 "sun" above (huǒ) 火 "fire." I think jiǒng originally meant "firelight," but I am currently referring to it as "warmth." It is interesting that the text does not use (rè) 熱 "heat" or (shǔ) 暑 "summerheat" or (huǒ) 火 "fire" or (wēn) 溫 "warm," but 炅.

Five colors visual diagnosis and vessel palpation

The Emperor says, "We have spoken of what is comprehensible. What about seeing what is visible?" Qi Bo gives him a basic visual diagnosis via 5 Colors: Yellow/Red = Heat, White = Cold, Green/Black = Pain.

"And palpating the tangible?"

Qi Bo says, "The vessels mainly affected are hard with blood and sunken; they may all be palpated."

Effects of emotion on qi movement

Emotion/Qi movement	Explanation
怒則氣上 (nù zé qì shàng) Anger makes qi rise	Qi counterflows[115]
喜則氣緩 (xǐ zé qì huǎn) Joy makes qi slow	Qi is harmonious. Willpower arrives. Nutritive and defensive qi flow smoothly
悲則氣消 (bēi zé qì xiāo) Sadness makes qi wasted	Heart contracts. Lung leaves rise upward, which leads to upper jiāo congestion, AKA nutritive and defensive qi are not dispersing, creating *Heat* (i.e. trapped yang qi) which consumes qi
恐則氣下 (kǒng zé qì xià) Fear makes qi descend	Jīng-essence retreats. Upper jiāo closes. Qi returning downward leads to lower jiāo distension
寒則氣收 (hán zé qì shōu) Cold makes qi contract	Interstices are closed, qi does not move
炅則氣泄 (jiǒng zé qì xiè) Warmth makes qi leak	Interstices open, profuse sweating ensues
驚則氣亂 (jīng zé qì luàn) Shock makes qi chaotic	Heart has nothing to lean on. Shén-spirit has nothing to return to. Anxieties have no anchor
勞則氣耗 (láo zé qì hào) Exertion makes qi spent	Wheezing, panting, and sweating lead to overextending, both externally and internally
思則氣結 (sī zé qì jié) Thought makes qi knotted	Heart conserves. Shén-spirit returns. Upright qi stays and does not move

Discussion on Abdomen and Middle

腹中論

(fù zhōng lùn)

Chapter 40, Discussion on Abdomen and Middle, introduces a number of internal conditions with fascinating treatment suggestions, such as chicken feces for *Drum Distension*, cuttlefish bone with sparrow egg and madder root* for *Blood Withering* or *Hidden Beam*, the pathogenesis and recurrence of *Heat Stroke*, *Wasting Center*, and *Reversal Counterflow*, and how to differentiate all of the above from plain old pregnancy.

---

* 蘆茹 (lǘ rú): an alternate name for 茜草根 (qiàn cǎo gēn).

Diseases mentioned in Chapter 40

Presentation	Name	Treatment (Taboos)
Heart/Abdomen fullness, can eat at dawn but not at dusk	*Drum Distension* 鼓脹 (gǔ zhàng)	
	Blood Withering 血枯 (xiě kū)	
	Hidden [Roof] Beam 伏梁 (fú liáng)	
	Heat Stroke 熱中 (rè zhòng) *Wasting Center* 消中 (xiāo zhōng)	**Minerals** create *Abscess*[116] 瘨 (chēn) **Aromatic herbs** create *Mania* 狂 (kuáng)
Breast swelling, neck pain, chest fullness, abdominal distension	*Reversal Counterflow* 厥逆 (jué nì)	**Moxibustion** creates *Aphonia* 瘖 (yīn) **Stone** creates *Mania* 狂 (kuáng)
Body has symptoms but no disease pulse	*Pregnancy* 懷子 (huái zǐ)	
Heat with pain	*Bloating Distension* 䐜脹 (chēn zhàng) *Headache* 頭痛 (tóu tòng)	

Pricking Low Back Pain

刺腰痛

(cì yāo tòng)

I vaguely remember trying to read Chapter 41 because the title is so straightforward, Pricking Low Back Pain, which sounds useful for a newly licensed acupuncturist practicing in the US today, where every doctor thinks "low back pain!" when considering acupuncture as a referral option. However, most of the suggestions are for bloodletting acupoints/channels we did not learn, or perhaps locations I should know by another name.

Points for low back pain

Low back pain of	Symptoms	Prick
Foot Taiyang 足太陽 (zú tài yáng)	Nape, spine, sacrum, back heavy	Bleed Taiyang channel center of knee (UB40)
Shaoyang 少陽 (shào yáng)	Difficult flexion/extension, lateral rotation	Bleed Shaoyang end of fibula (GB34)
Yangming 陽明 (yáng míng)	Difficult lateral rotation, sees [ghosts] if laterally rotated, sad	Yangming before the upper tibia (St36) 3 (wěi) 痏[117]
Foot Shaoyin 足少陰 (zú shào yīn)	Radiates into inner spine	Shaoyin above inner malleolus (K7) 2 (wěi) 痏

Jueyin 厥陰 (jué yīn)	Like drawn bow, talkative, unintelligible	Jueyin vessel between calf and Achilles tendon (Lv5) 2 (wěi) 痏
Separator Vessel* 解脈 (jiě mài)	Radiates to shoulders, blurry vision, incontinence	Bleed outer border of popliteal sinew and muscle (UB39) until blood changes
Separator Vessel 解脈 (jiě mài) with 帶 (dài)†	Low back feels broken, fearful	Bleed UB40 grain-like varicosities until black blood turns red
Same Yin‡ 同陰 (tóng yīn)	As if small hammers reside within, sudden swelling	Above outer malleolus at end of fibula (GB39) 3 (wěi) 痏
Yang Linking 陽維 (yáng wéi)	Sudden swelling	Yangwei/Taiyang meeting point on calf ~ 1 尺 (chǐ)§ off the ground (UB57)
Belt Vessel¶ 衡絡 (héng luò)	Difficult flexion/extension, fear of falling in extension, caused by heavy lifting injury	Bleed between sinews of the popliteal [crease] (K10 and UB39?)
Meeting Yin 會陰 (huì yīn)**	Pain causes profuse sweating, followed by thirst with desire to drink, and a desire to walk	5 cùn above qiào (UB56)
Fly [and] Soar 飛揚 (fēi yáng)††	As if blown by wind, sad and fearful	Yangwei meeting point; luò-connecting point of Foot Taiyang (UB58)
Prosperous Yang 昌陽 (chāng yáng)‡‡	Radiates to pectorals, blurry vision, in extreme cases aphasic	2 cùn above medial malleolus, anterior to the sinew and posterior to Taiyin (K7)

---

* 解脈 (jiě mài) Separator Vessel: most commentaries place this as a branch of the Foot Taiyang channel.

† This may not be the 帶脈 (dài mài) Belt Vessel but the sensation of a belt pulled tight.

‡ 同陰 (tóng yīn): most commentaries place this as a branch of the Foot Shaoyang.

§ 尺 (chǐ): unit of measurement equal to 10 (cùn) 寸.

¶ 橫絡 (héng luò) "Horizontal Collateral" is an alternate name for the Belt Vessel.

** **Acu Trivia!** 會陰 (huì yīn) "Meeting Yin" is the name of R1.

†† **Acu Trivia!** 飛揚 (fēi yáng) "Fly [and] Soar" is the name of UB58.

‡‡ **Acu Trivia!** 昌陽 (chāng yáng) "Prosperous Yang" is an alternate name of K7.

Scatter? 散 (sǎn)*	Hot, vexatious, as if a horizontal wood resides within, extreme cases incontinent	Crevice between bone and flesh in front of the knee
Flesh Lining 肉里 (ròu lǐ)†	Cannot cough, cough causes sinews to cramp acutely	Behind GB39 outside the Taiyang (possibly GB38)

The last paragraph is somewhat useful if you know all the channels by their 6 channels designation (e.g. Foot Shaoyin).

Channels for low back pain

Low back pain	Needle
Along spine up to head dizzy, vision blurry, tends to fall	Bleed Foot Taiyang (UB40)
Upper cold	Foot Taiyang/Yangming
Upper heat	Foot Jueyin
Inability to flex/extend	Foot Shaoyang
Center heat with shortness of breath	Foot Shaoyin, bleed UB40
Upper cold with inability to laterally rotate	Foot Yangming
Upper heat [with inability to laterally rotate]	Foot Taiyin
Center heat with shortness of breath	Foot Shaoyin
Constipation	Foot Shaoyin
Lower abdominal fullness	Foot Jueyin
As if [back is] broken, inability to flex/extend/lift	Foot Taiyang
Radiates to inner spine	Foot Shaoyin
Radiates to lower and lateral abdomen with inability to extend spine	Lumbar/Sacrum meeting [area] above PSIS (posterior superior iliac spine) and gluteals

Needle right for left, left for right (i.e. contralaterally).

---

*   According to Wang Bing, 散 (sǎn) is a branch of the Spleen channel.

†   According to Wang Bing, 肉里 (ròu lǐ) is related to the Shaoyang and Yangwei. Other commentators are unsure.

Discussion on Wind

風論

(fēng lùn)

Chapter 42, Discussion on Wind, discusses several diseases.

(hán rè) 寒熱 *Cold Heat*

Etiology: wind is hiding between the skin, opening and closing the pores[100]

Presentation/Pathogenesis: sudden chills from open interstices leads to poor appetite; hot and stifled [sensation] from closed interstices leads to muscle wasting

(rè zhòng) 熱中 *Heat Stroke*

Etiology: wind qi travels into Stomach through Yangming up to inner canthus, patient overweight so qi cannot escape outward

Presentation: eyes yellow

(hán zhōng) 寒中 *Cold Stroke*

Etiology: wind qi travels into Stomach through Yangming up to inner canthus, patient underweight, therefore outward leakage leads to cold

Presentation: tears exit (i.e. watery eyes)

(lì fēng) 癘風 *Pestilential Wind* *

Etiology: wind qi enters back-shū points through Taiyang and disrupts the defensive qi	Nutritive qi hot rot
Presentation: muscle bloating/ulcers, numbness	Bridge of nose, complexion, and skin ulcerative erosions

(piān kū) 偏枯 *Asymmetrical Withering*†
Different types of *Wind* mentioned in Chapter 42

Pattern	Pathogenesis
	Presentation
Liver Wind 肝風 (gān fēng)	Contracted in spring
	Profuse sweating, averse to wind, easily sad or angry, complexion slightly green, throat dry, occasionally abhors women (i.e. no libido?), blue-green bags below eyes
Heart Wind 心風 (xīn fēng)	Contracted in summer
	Profuse sweating, averse to wind, easily angry or frightened, complexion red, mouth red. In extreme cases, cannot speak quickly
Spleen Wind 脾風 (pí fēng)	Contracted in (jì xià) 季夏 "last-month-of summer" longsummer?
	Profuse sweating, averse to wind, body loose, feels exhausted and does not want to move, complexion sallow, poor appetite, nose yellow

---

* "Wind-Cold lodged in vessels can be named *Pestilential Wind* or *Cold Heat.*" *Pestilential Wind* is leprosy.

† Mentioned in first paragraph, but does not recur for the rest of the chapter. Maybe *Asymmetrical Withering*, aka hemiplegia, is related to *Wind*?

Lung Wind 肺風 (fèi fēng)	Contracted in autumn
	Profuse sweating, averse to wind, complexion white, occasional cough or shortness of breath that is better in daytime, worse at night, brow white
Kidney Wind 腎風 (shèn fēng)	Contracted in winter
	Profuse sweating, averse to wind, face puffy, spine pain with inability to stand straight, complexion sooty, difficulty with flexion and extension, muscles black
Stomach Wind 胃風 (wèi fēng)	No pathogenesis mentioned
	Profuse sweating on neck, averse to wind, inability to eat or drink, congestion in diaphragm, frequent abdominal bloating, diarrhea if cold foods eaten, body thin but belly large
Asymmetrical Wind[101] 偏風 (piān fēng)	Contracted when wind attacks the corresponding back-shū points
	No presentation mentioned
Brain Wind 腦風 (nǎo fēng)	Contracted when wind enters Du16
	No presentation mentioned
Eye Wind 目風 (mù fēng)	Contracted when wind enters head
	Eyes cold
Leaking Wind 漏風 (lòu fēng)	Contracted from drinking alcohol
	Profuse sweating, need to wear layers, sweat after eating, in extreme cases: body sweats, short of breath, averse to wind, clothes often soggy, mouth dry, thirsty, unable to exert self
Internal Wind 內風 (nèi fēng)	Contracted from sweating during sex
	No presentation mentioned
Head Wind 首風 (shǒu fēng)	Contracted just after bathing
	Profuse sweat on head and face, averse to wind, unrelenting headache if exposed to wind
Diarrhea Wind 泄風 (xiè fēng)	Chronic wind enters the middle [jiāo] and lodges in interstices
	Profuse sweat dampens clothes, mouth dry, upper body looks marinated [in sweat], unable to exert self, whole body pain with cold [sensation]
Intestinal Wind 腸風 (cháng fēng)	Chronic wind enters the middle jiāo
	Undigested food in stools

Chapter 43

Discussion on Impediment

痹論

(bì lùn)

Chapter 43, Discussion on Impediment, goes through all the categorizations of (bì) 痹 *Impediment*. It begins with the three types caused by external pathological factors that I learned in acupuncture school as a student.

External impediments

Disease	Etiology
Moving Impediment 行痹 (xíng bì)	Wind
Painful Impediment 痛痹 (tòng bì)	Cold
Fixed Impediment 着痹 (zhuó bì)	Damp

Impediments that correspond to the seasons and the Zang

	Contracted in	Damages ~ if untreated
Bone Impediment 骨痹 (gǔ bì)	Winter 冬 (dōng)	Kidney 腎 (shèn)
Sinew Impediment 筋痹 (jīn bì)	Spring 春 (chūn)	Liver 肝 (gān)
Vessel Impediment 脈痹 (mài bì)	Summer 夏 (xià)	Heart 心 (xīn)
Muscle Impediment 肌痹 (jī bì)	Ultimate Yin 至陰 (zhì yīn)	Spleen 脾 (pí)
Skin Impediment 皮痹 (pí bì)	Autumn 秋 (qiū)	Lung 肺 (fèi)

There are neat little descriptions of what each Zang's *Impediment* looks like. There is also (in addition to the Five Zang Bi) Intestinal Bi and Uterus Bi.

Condition	Symptoms
Lung Impediment 肺痹 (fèi bì)	Vexation, fullness, panting and retching
Heart Impediment 心痹 (xīn bì)	Vessel stoppage, vexation and distension in epigastrium, violent upward qi followed by panting, dry throat, hiccups, reversal qi creates fear
Liver Impediment 肝痹 (gān bì)	Startle at night when sleeping, drink copiously, frequent urination, upper [body] like drawn bow or pregnant
Kidney Impediment 腎痹 (shèn bì)	Tendency for distension, sacrum for heel (i.e. want to squat/sit all the time), spine for head (i.e. severe kyphosis)
Spleen Impediment 脾痹 (pí bì)	Four limbs loose and lazy, cough and retch liquid (i.e. productive cough), large congestion above (i.e. glomus)
Intestinal Impediment 腸痹 (cháng bì)	Frequent drinking but [urine] inhibited, borborygmus, occasional undigested food in stools
Uterus Impediment 胞痹 (bāo bì)	Lower abdomen and bladder tender to palpation as if soaked in hot water, inhibited urination, clear nasal discharge

I am not quite sure how the next two sentences relate to the topic of the chapter, but as a standalone statement they do make sense:

陰氣者，靜則神藏，躁則消亡。

(yīn qì zhě, jìng zé shén cáng, zào zé xiāo wáng)

Yin qi conserves in the spirit when quiet, perishes when restless.

飲食自倍，腸胃乃傷。

(yǐn shí zì bèi, cháng wèi nǎi shāng)

Multiple portions of food and drink harms the gut and the stomach.

Impediment symptoms

Symptom	Impediment in
Audible panting	Lung
Worry and over-thinking	Heart
Incontinence	Kidney
Unquenchable thirst	Liver
Muscle vanishing	Spleen

Impediment prognoses

If Impediment	Consequence
Enters Zang	Death
Lingers between sinews and bones	Chronic pain
Lingers in skin and muscle	Easy to cure

The Emperor inquires about the six Fu, and Qi Bo explains that *Impediment* enters the Zang via hé-sea points, the Fu via back-shū points. The Emperor then inquires about the nutritive and defensive qi. Qi Bo answers with a description of the nature of defensive qi and concludes, "Because it cannot combine with wind, cold, or damp, [wei qi] *Impediment* does not occur."

Etiology of symptoms

Symptom	Etiology
Pain	More cold qi
No pain, numbness	Long-standing condition that has entered deeply, wei qi does not flow well through the channels so poor circulation ensues
Cold	Less yang qi, more yin qi
Symptom	Etiology
Heat	More yang qi, less yin qi
Profuse sweating and sogginess	Extreme dampness, less yang qi, abundant yin qi

Painless impediments

Symptom	Impediment at
Heaviness	Bone
No blood circulation	Vessel
Cramp	Sinew
Numbness	Flesh
Cold	Skin

Discussion on Atrophy

痿論

(wěi lùn)

Chapter 44, Discussion on Atrophy, discusses how the five Zang cause lameness.

Types of atrophy

Zang	Governs	Heat[102] in said Zang causes	Condition
Lung	Skin Body-hair	Skin deficiency and dryness	*Atrophy Lameness* 痿躄 (wěi bì)
Heart	Blood Vessels	Upward reversal, which creates deficiency below	*Vessel Atrophy* 脈痿 (mài wěi)[103]
Liver	Sinews Membranes	Gallbladder leakage (mouth bitter, sinews and membranes dry), which creates cramping	*Sinew Atrophy* 筋痿 (jīn wěi)
Spleen	Muscle Flesh	Stomach dryness, thirst, muscle numbness	*Flesh Atrophy* 肉痿 (ròu wěi)
Kidney	Bone Marrow	Lumbar/Spine inability to lift, bones wither and marrow decreases	*Bone Atrophy* 骨痿 (gǔ wěi)

The Emperor asks Qi Bo to expand on the pathophysiology of each type of atrophy. In reply, Qi Bo refers to two books called *Běn Bìng* 《本病》 <u>Root of Disease</u>, and *Xià Jīng* 《下經》 <u>Lower Classic</u>.*

(wěi bì) 痿躄 *Atrophy Lameness*

Lung is the eldest of the Zang, and the lid of Heart. If Lung is distressed it will make sounds, indicating that the Lung leaves† are dry due to heat

Differentiation: Lung heat, complexion white, body-hair falls out

(mài wěi) 脈痿 *Vessel Atrophy*

Excess sadness causes the (bāo luò jué) 胞絡 Uterus Collateral Vanishing, which moves yang qi internally, expressing (xīn xià bēng) 心下崩 *Epigastric Avalanche* and frequent hematuria. Thus <u>Root of Disease</u> states, "Large channels that are empty generate (jī bì) 肌痹 *Muscle Impediment*, which spreads to become (mài wěi) 脈痿 *Vessel Atrophy*"

Differentiation: Heart heat, complexion red, collateral vessels overflow

(jīn wěi) 筋痿 *Sinew Atrophy*

Endless thinking and longing for that which one cannot have, intention spilled out, [and/or] too much sex loosens the (zōng jīn) 宗筋 "ancestral sinew," a euphemism for the penis. Thus <u>Lower Classic</u> states, "*Sinew Atrophy* occurs from Liver exerting within"

Differentiation: Liver heat, complexion bluish-gray, nails wither

(ròu wěi) 肉痿 *Flesh Atrophy*

Proximity to damp, working in water, or living in damp conditions, the muscles become soggy and marinated, impeded and numb. Thus the <u>Lower Classic</u> states, "*Flesh Atrophy* occurs [in] damp places"

Differentiation: Spleen heat, complexion yellow, flesh twitches involuntarily

---

* We have not seen references to other books since Chapters 15 and 19.

† Leaves: plural of leaf. The lungs were shaped like a tree in Chinese anatomy.

(gǔ wěi) 骨痿 *Bone Atrophy*

Distant travel, labor to exhaustion, thirst from great heat, the thirst consumes yang qi from within, and heat lodges in Kidney. Kidney is a water organ; when water does not control fire, the bones wither and marrow becomes deficient, the feet do not respond to the body['s commands]. Thus <u>Lower Classic</u> states, "*Bone Atrophy* comes of great heat"

Differentiation: Kidney heat, complexion black, teeth rot

Treating *Atrophy* with Yangming

The last paragraph of Chapter 44 explains why it is possible to treat *Atrophy* using only Yangming points. "Yangming is the sea of five Zang and six Fu; it governs the ancestral tendon. The ancestral tendon is responsible for bundling bones* and lubricating joints. The (chōng mài) 沖脈 Penetrating Vessel is the sea of channels and vessels; it governs irrigating the streams and valleys, and converges† with Yangming at the ancestral tendon, meeting at St30‡ with Yangming as the elder. They all belong to the (dài mài) 帶脈 Belt Vessel and network with the (dū mài) 督脈 Governing Vessel. Therefore, when Yangming is deficient, the ancestral tendon is flaccid, the Belt Vessel does not contract, and the legs atrophy into dysfunction... Treat by tonifying the yíng-spring and clearing the back-shū."

---

*   **Acu Trivia!** 束骨 (shù gǔ) "Bundle Bone" is the name of UB65.

†   A note on the verb *converge*: this is the same character (hé) 合 as in hé-sea point, which I believe would be better translated as hé-convergent point, because it is where the (wèi qì) 衛氣 leaves the surface and goes deep inside to converge with the (yuán qì) 元氣.

‡   **Acu Trivia!** 氣街 (qì jiē) is an alternate name for 氣衝 (qì chōng), St30, where the Chong Mai begins.

Discussion on Reversal

厥論

(jué lùn)

Chapter 45, Discussion on Reversal, divides (jué) 厥 *Reversal*
into two main types, cold and hot.

(hán jué) 寒厥 *Cold Reversal*

Etiology: yang qi deficient below	Onset: toes to top of knee cold
Pathophysiology: Yin qi originates in the interior of the five toes, gathers below the knee and accumulates above the knee. Yang qi is injured and unable to seep and fill the channels and collaterals. Yin qi alone remains; therefore, the hands and feet are cold	

(rè jué) 熱厥 *Heat Reversal*

Etiology: Yin qi deficient below	Onset: soles of feet hot
Pathophysiology: yang qi originates in the exterior of the five toes, gathers in the soles of the foot and accumulates at K1 for patients with strong constitutions who overindulge in sex in the autumn and winter,[104] whose lower qi ascends and cannot return, jing-essence and qi leak downward, and evil qi ascends. Alcohol enters Stomach, filling the collaterals and emptying the channels. Spleen is responsible for moving the fluids for Stomach. When yin qi is deficient, then yang qi enters. When yang qi enters, then Stomach is not harmonious. When Stomach is not harmonious, then jing-essence and qi are depleted. When jing-essence is depleted, it cannot nourish the four limbs. Such a patient must frequently engage in sexual activity when intoxicated. Qi gathers in the Spleen and cannot disperse; alcohol and grain qi clash with each other, creating abundant heat in the middle; therefore, there is internal heat and dark urine	

This is a great passage on how alcohol metabolizes in the body from a Chinese medicine perspective. Qi Bo adds, "Alcohol has abundant and fierce qi. If the Kidney qi is frail, and yang qi alone is present, the hands and feet feel hot."

Diagnosis clarifications

Abdominal fullness	Yin qi abundant above and deficient below
Sudden inability to recognize people	Yang qi abundant above, lower qi counterflows upward, creating chaos

Manifestations of *Reversal*

Reversal of	Manifestations
Jùyáng	*Swollen Head* 腫首 (zhǒng shǒu) *Head Heavy* 頭重 (tóu zhòng) *Inability to Walk* 足不能行 (zú bù néng xíng) *Episodes of Syncope* 眴仆 (xún pū)
Yangming	*Vertex Disease* 巔疾 (diān jí) *Desire to Run and Shout* 欲走呼 (yù zǒu hū) *Abdominal Fullness* 腹滿 (fù mǎn) *Inability to Fall Asleep* 不得臥 (bù dé wò) *Face Red and Hot* 面赤而熱 (miàn chì ér rè) *Hallucinations and Ravings* 妄見而妄言 (wàng jiàn ér wàng yán)
Shaoyang	*Violent Deafness* 暴聾 (bào lóng) *Cheeks Swollen and Hot* 頰腫而熱 (jiá zhǒng ér rè) *Rib Pain* 脇痛 (xié tòng) *Lower Legs Cannot Transport* 胻不可以運 (héng bù kě yǐ yùn)
Taiyin	*Abdominal Fullness* 腹滿 (fù mǎn) *Bloating Distension* 䐜脹 (chēn zhàng) *Constipation* 後不利 (hòu bú lì) *Low Appetite* 不欲食 (bú yù shí) *Retching After Eating* 食則嘔 (shí zé ǒu) *Inability to Fall Asleep* 不得臥 (bù dé wò)
Shaoyin	*Dry Mouth* 口乾 (kǒu gān) *Urine red* 溺赤 (nìao chì) *Abdominal Fullness* 腹滿 (fù mǎn) *Heart Pain* 心痛 (xīn tòng)
Jueyin	*Hypogastric Swelling and Pain* 少腹腫痛 (shào fù zhǒng tòng) *Abdominal Distension* 腹脹 (fù zhàng) *Inhibited Urination* 涇溲不利 (jīng sōu bú lì) *Prefers Lying Down with Knees Bent* 好臥屈膝 (hào wò qū xī) *Genitals Retract and/or Swell* 陰縮腫 (yīn suō zhǒng) *Lower Legs Internal Heat* 胻內熱 (héng nèi rè)

Treatment: Drain excess and tonify deficiency. If neither excess nor deficient, take the jīng-river.

Reversal Counterflow[105] of	Symptoms/Prognosis
Taiyin	*Acute Lower Leg Cramps* 胻急攣 (héng jí luán) *Heart Pain Radiating to Abdomen* 心痛引腹 (xīn tòng yǐn fù)
Shaoyin	*Deficient Fullness* 虛滿 (xū mǎn) *Retching Change* 嘔變 (ǒu biàn) *Diarrhea Clear* 下泄清 (xià xiè qīng)
Jueyin	*Cramping* 攣 (luán) *Low Back Pain* 腰痛 (yāo tòng) *Deficient Fullness* 虛滿 (xū mǎn) *Frontal Block*, i.e. urinary blockage 前閉 (qián bì) *Delirious Speech* 譫言 (zhān yán)
All 3 yins	*Fecal and Urinary Blockage* 不得前後 (bù dé qián hòu) *Hands and Feet Cold* 手足寒 (shǒu zú hán) Death in 3 days
Taiyang	*Stiff Syncope* 僵仆 (jiāng pū) *Retch Blood*, i.e. Hematemesis 嘔血 (ǒu xiě) *Tendency for Nosebleed* 善衄 (shàn nù)
Shaoyang	*Joints Inarticulate*, i.e. low back unable to move, neck unable to laterally rotate 機關不利 (jī guān bú lì) If expressed as (yáng yōng) 陽癰 *Yang Carbuncle*, untreatable If (jīng) 驚 *Shock*, death
Yangming	*Panting Cough* 喘欬 (chuǎn ké) *Body Hot* 身熱 (shēn rè) Tendency for (jīng) 驚 *Shock*, (nù) 衄 *Nosebleed*, and (ǒu xiě) 嘔血 *Hematemesis*
Hand Taiyin	*Deficient Fullness with Cough* 虛滿而欬 (xū mǎn ér ké) *Tendency to Retch Foam* 善嘔沫 (shàn ǒu mò)
Hand Jueyin[106]	*Heart Pain Radiating to Throat* 心痛引喉 (xīn tòng yǐn hóu) *Body Hot* 身熱 (shēn rè) [indicates] death, cannot be treated
Hand Taiyang	*Deafness* 耳聾 (ěr lóng) *Tears Exude* 泣出 (qì chū) *Nape Cannot Laterally Rotate* 項不可以顧 (xiàng bù kě yǐ gù) *Low Back Cannot Flex/Extend* 腰不可以俛仰 (yāo bù kě yǐ fǔ yǎng)
Hand Yangming/ Shaoyang	*Throat Impediment* 喉痹 (hóu bì) *Esophagus Swelling* 嗌腫 (yì zhǒng) *Tetany* 痓 (zhì)

Discussion on Disease Capabilities

病能論

(bìng néng lùn)

Chapter 46, Discussion on Disease Capabilities, answers a series of questions the Emperor poses on the following diseases.

(wèi wǎn yōng) 胃脘癰 *Stomach Ulcer*

Diagnosis: Stomach pulse should be deep and thin, indicating (qì nì) 氣逆 *Qi Counterflow*. For *Counterflow*, the carotid pulse should be excessive, indicating *Heat*. St9 is the Stomach pulse

Etiology: *Counterflow* and excess indicates *Heat* accumulating inside and not moving out of the Stomach

(wò bù ān) 臥不安 *Restless Sleep*, i.e. waking often

Etiology: Zang injury, jīng-essence has nowhere to abide

(bù dé yǎn wò) 不得偃臥 *Inability to Sleep Supine*

Etiology: Lung is the cover for the Zang. If Lung qi is excess then pulse is large

(jué) 厥 *Reversal*

Pulse: deep tight right, floating slow left

Diagnosis: in winter, the right pulse should be deep tight—this reflects the season. The left pulse is floating slow—this is counter to the season. Left indicates disease at Kidney, relating to Lung. [The patient should have] low back pain

Etiology: Shaoyin Vessel runs through Kidney and networks Lung. Getting a Lung pulse texture indicates Kidney disease, therefore there should be low back pain relating to Kidney

(jǐng yōng) 頸癰 *Neck Ulcer*

Question: Why can this be cured by stone, needling, or moxibustion?

Answer: Ulcers are best excised by needling open. Qi and blood accumulation are best drained by stone.*

(yáng jué) 陽厥 *Yang Reversal*

Symptoms: rage, mania

Pulse: Yangming (dòng) 動 "moves" Juyang Shaoyang (bú dòng) 不動 "does not move"

Etiology: yang qi when violently cut off leads to irritability. Food enters yin and feeds qi to yang

Treatment: no food, drink (shēng tiě luò) 生鐵洛 "raw iron chippings" to descend qi

(jiǔ fēng) 酒風 *Alcohol Wind*

Symptoms: body hot and indolent, sweating as if in a bath, aversion to wind, shortness of breath

---

*   This is known as (tóng bìng yì zhì) 同病異治 "same disease, different treatment"

Treatment: take 10 fēn[107] (zé xiè) 澤瀉, 10 fēn (zhú) 朮,[108] 5 fēn (lù xián cǎo) 鹿銜草. A pinch with 3 fingers before meals

The last few sentences summarize the ethics of practicing acupuncture and the contents of five books lost to history.

Five books lost to history

Title	Contents
Shàng Jīng 《上經》 Upper Classic	On how qi connects to the sky (i.e. weather)
Xià Jīng 《下經》 Lower Classic	On how disease conditions change and transform
Jīn Guì 《金匱》 Golden Cabinet*	On death and life (i.e. prognosis)
Kuí Duó 《揆度》 Formulas and Pulses	On herbal formulas and pulse taking
Qí Héng 《奇恆》 Extraordinary Prognoses	On extraordinary diseases and seasonal prognoses

---

*   Not to be confused with Zhāng Zhòngjǐng's *Jīn Guì Yào Luè* 《金匱要略》 Essentials of the Golden Cabinet.

Discussion on Extraordinary Diseases

奇病論

(qí bìng lùn)

Chapter 47, Discussion on Extraordinary Diseases, contains another list of unusual conditions. Here are a few of them.

(bāo luò jué) 胞絡絕 *Uterus Collateral Extinction*

Symptoms: body heavy, lose voice in September
Etiology: Uterus Collateral is fastened to the Kidney Shaoyin Vessel, goes through the Kidney and connects to the root of the tongue
Treatment: not necessary, will regain voice in October

(xī jī) 息積 *Breath Accumulation*

Symptoms: hypochondriac fullness with counterflow qi for 2–3 years
Treatment: no moxibustion or acupuncture, use exercise in conjunction with herbs

(fú liáng) 伏梁 *Hidden Roofbeam*

Symptoms: thighs, buttocks, and calves swollen, navel pain

Etiology: wind qi overflows into LI, dwells in membranes below

Treatment: do not move, otherwise urinary incontinence and inhibition may occur

(zhěn jīn) 疹筋 *Papule Sinew*

Symptoms: extremely rapid chi pulse, sinews cramp, abdominal cramps; white/black color appears in extreme cases

(jué nì) 厥逆 *Reversal Counterflow*

Symptoms: headache that lasts many years, teeth also hurt

Etiology: great cold enters the bone marrow, creating counterflow in the brain

(pí dān) 脾癉 *Spleen Drought*

Symptoms: mouth dry, internal heat, fullness in the middle

Etiology: overeating, fats, sweets

Pathophysiology: five qi overflows upward, can develop into (xiāo kě) 消渴 *Thirsting and Wasting*

Treatment: use (lán) 蘭 "orchid"[109] to eliminate (chén) 陳 "aged"[110] qi

(dǎn dān) 膽癉 *Gallbladder Drought*

Symptoms: bitter taste in mouth

Etiology: Liver is the general of the middle who makes decisions according to the Gallbladder; the throat is its envoy. Repeated strategizing without decision leads to deficient Gallbladder qi overflowing upward

Treatment: (yáng líng quán) 陽陵泉 GB34, (dǎn mù) 膽募 GB24, (dǎn shū) 膽俞 UB19

Five excesses and two insufficiences

(wǔ yǒu jú) 五有餘 five excesses	(èr bù zú) 二不足 two insufficiencies
Symptoms: body hot as embers, neck and chest (gé) 格 Repel, i.e. continuous vomiting	(lóng) 癃 *Urine Retention*, frequent urination (20+ times/day), pulse faint and thin as a hair
Prognosis: death	

(tāi bìng) 胎病 *Congenital Seizures*

Symptoms: born with (diān jí) 巔疾 *Vertex Disease*

Etiology: mother experienced great (jīng) 驚 *Shock* while pregnant, qi ascends and does not descend, jīng-essence and qi dwell together, therefore her child has (diān jí) 巔疾 *Vertex Disease*

(shèn fēng) 腎風 *Kidney Wind*

Symptom: sudden *Water* [signs], very tight pulse but no pain, no wasting but unable to eat, low appetite

Etiology: Kidney

Pathophysiology: tendency for (jīng) 驚 *Shock*, if Heart qi atrophies [patient will] die

Discussion on the Great Extraordinaries

大奇論

(dà qí lùn)

Chapter 48, Discussion on the Great Extraordinaries, foregoes the question-and-answer format and is simply a list.

Pulse images and diseases from Chapter 48

Zang	Pulse	Signs and symptoms		
Lung	Full and solid	*Swelling* 腫 (zhǒng)	*Bilateral Torso Fullness* 兩胠滿 (liǎng qū mǎn)	*Panting* 喘 (chuǎn)
Liver			*Startle Awake* 臥則驚 (wò zé jīng)	
			Inability to Urinate 不得小便 (bù dé xiǎo biàn)	
Kidney			Soles to hypogastrium full Calves change sizes Hip/Knee-related limp with tendency for *Asymmetrical Withering*, aka hemiplegia 偏枯 (piān kū)	

Heart	Full and large	*Seizures* 癇 (xián) *Convulsions* 瘛 (chì) *Sinew Cramps* 筋攣 (jīn luán)	
Liver	Small urgent		
Liver	Galloping violently	*Shock Terrors*[111] 驚駭 (jīng hài)	
Kidney	Small urgent, not drum	*Conglomeration* 瘕 (jiǎ)	
Liver			
Heart			
Kidney and Liver (both)	Deep	*Stone Water* 石水 (shí shuǐ)	
	Floating	*Wind Water* 風水 (fēng shuǐ)	
	Empty	Death	
	Small wiry	*Imminent Shock* 欲驚 (yù jīng)	
Kidney	Large urgent Deep	*Hernia* 疝 (shàn)	
Liver			
Heart	Wide slippery Urgent	*Heart Hernia* 心疝 (xīn shàn) aka Running Piglet	
Lung	Deep wide	*Lung Hernia* 肺疝 (fèi shàn)	
3 yang	Urgent	*Conglomeration* 瘕 (jiǎ)	
3 yin		*Hernia* 疝 (shàn)	
2 yin		*Seizure Reversal* 癇厥 (xián jué)	
2 yang		*Shock* 驚 (jīng)	
Spleen	Drums outward Deep	*Intestinal Blockage* 腸癖 (cháng pǐ)	Will gradually resolve on its own
Liver	Small Moderate		Easy to treat
Kidney	Small wide Deep	*Hematochezia* 下血 (xià xiě)	If blood is warm and body is hot, death

Zang	Pulse	Signs and symptoms
Heart		*Blockage* 癖 (pǐ) with *Hematochezia* 下血 (xià xiě)
Liver		Treatable if both Zang affected If body is hot, death [occurs] 7 days from *Heat* signs
Stomach	Deep drum Choppy large	*Hemiplegia* 偏枯 (piān kū) Males express left, females express right. Treatable if there is no *Aphonia* 瘖 (yīn), recovery within 30 days. If there is *Aphonia* 瘖 (yīn), recovery within 3 years. If [patient is] younger than 20, die within 3 years
Heart	Small hard Urgent	

More pulse textures from Chapter 48

If pulse arrives wide with (xiě nǜ) 血衄 *Nosebleed* and (shēn rè) 身熱 *Body Hot*, patient will die
If pulse comes suspended hooked floating, that is normal
If pulse arrives as if panting, that is (bào jué) 暴厥 *Violent Reversal*[112]
If pulse arrives rapid, creating (bào jīng) 暴驚 *Violent Shock*, it will resolve itself in 3–4 days

Death pulse prognoses

Pulse arrives	Condition	Prognosis
Floating convergent rapid (more than 10 beats per breath)	Channel qi insufficiency	If faint, die in 90 days
Like fire catching (rú huǒ xīn rán) 如火薪然	Heart jīng-essence being granted [and/or] robbed	Die when grass dries
Like scattered leaves (sǎn yè) 散葉	Liver qi deficient	Die when tree leaves fall
Like questioning guests[113] (xǐng kè) 省客	Kidney qi insufficiency	Die if [pulse] goes suspended and jujubes are flourishing
Like pills of mud (wán ní) 丸泥	Stomach jīng-essence insufficiency	Die when elm pods fall
Like horizontal block (héng gé) 橫格	Gallbladder qi insufficiency	Die when rice ripens

Like wire filaments (xián lǚ) 弦縷	Uterus jīng-essence insufficiency	Verbose [patients] die when frost descends. Quiet [patients] can be cured
Like filtering lacquer* (jiāo qī) 交漆		If faint, die in 30 days
Like bubbling spring† (yǒng quán) 涌泉	Taiyang qi in muscle insufficiency	Die when chives blossom
Like ruined earth‡ (tuí tǔ) 頹土	Muscle qi insufficiency	Black/White complexion dies
Like suspended harmony§ (xuán yōng) 懸雍	12 back-shū insufficiency	Die when water freezes
Like upturned blade℄ (yǎn dāo) 偃刀	Cold Heat in Kidney	Die when spring begins**
Like pill†† (wán) 丸	Large Intestine qi insufficiency	Die when jujube leaves grow
Like magnificence‡‡ (huá) 華	Small Intestine qi insufficiency	Die in last month of autumn

---

* Filtering lacquer (jiāo qī) 交漆 pulse: arrives to the left and right sides [of where practitioner's fingers are pressing].

† Bubbling spring (yǒng quán) 涌泉 pulse: floating drum **Acu Trivia!** 涌泉 is the name of K1.

‡ Ruined Earth (tuí tǔ) 頹土 pulse: [practitioner applies] pressure and cannot find.

§ Suspended Harmony (xuán yōng) 懸雍 pulse: floating, also big.

℄ Upturned Blade (yǎn dāo) 偃刀 pulse: small and urgent in superficial, hard large and urgent in deeper levels.

** Solar Term! 立春 (lì chūn) "start of spring."

†† Pill (wán) 丸 pulse: slippery and cannot be felt in deeper levels.

‡‡ Magnificent (huá) 華 pulse: makes patient fearful, dislike sitting/lying down, listening often when walking/standing.

Pulse Explanations

脈解

(mài jiě)

Chapter 49, Pulse Explanations, goes through a lot of explanations by six channels (Taiyang, Shaoyang, Yangming, Taiyin, Shaoyin, Jueyin). There are many diseases mentioned, some of which I believe we have seen before.

Taiyang conditions mentioned in Chapter 49

Disease	Etiology
Swelling in Low Back 腫腰 (zhǒng yāo) *Coccyx Pain* 脽痛 *(shuí tòng)*	In the first month, yang qi comes out on top, yin qi abundant
Asymmetrical Deficiency 偏虛 (piān xū) leading to Limp 跛 (bǒ)	In the first month yang qi thaws and allows land qi come out
Stiffness Above 強上 (jiàng shàng) radiating to [upper] back	Yang qi rises up largely creating conflict above
Tinnitus 耳鳴 (ěr míng)	Yang qi makes all beings abundant and leap upwards

Mania 狂 (kuáng) *Vertex Disease* 巔疾 (diān jí)	Yang is all above, and yin qi follows below, creating deficiency below and excess above
Floating [pulse?] 浮 (fú) Leading to *Deafness* 聾 (lóng)	All at qi
Enters middle to become *Aphonia* 瘖 (yīn)	Yang abundance weakens
Internal Robbery 內奪 (nèi duó) Leading to *Reversal* 厥 (jué)[114]	Kidney deficiency

Shaoyang conditions mentioned in Chapter 49

Heart/Rib Pain 心脇痛 (xīn xié tòng)	Shaoyang abundant, in the ninth month yang qi ends and yin qi becomes abundant
Inability to Extend/Laterally Rotate 不可反側 (bù kě fǎn cè)	Yin qi hides substance, making it difficult to move
In extreme cases, *Jumps* 躍 (yuè)[115]	In the ninth month all things grow frail, grass and tree [leaves] fall, qi goes from yang to yin, abundance grows below

Yangming conditions mentioned in Chapter 49

Endless Shivering Chills 洒洒振寒 (sǎ sǎ zhèn hán)	The fifth month is the yin of abundant yang. Yang is abundant and yin qi is added atop it
Shin Swelling 脛腫 (jìng zhǒng) *Gluteals not Contracting* 股不收 (gǔ bù shōu)	The fifth month is the yin of abundant yang. A single yin ascends, beginning to conflict with yang
Upper Panting 上喘 (shàng chuǎn) leading to *Water* 水 (shuǐ)	Yin qi descends and re-ascends, pathogens lodge between Zang and Fu
Chest Pain 胸痛 (xiōng tòng) *Scant Qi* 少氣 (shǎo qì)	Water qi at Zang and Fu; water is yin
In extreme cases, *Reversal*, averse to people and fire, startled by the sound of wood	Yang and yin battle; water and fire averse to each other

Desires solitude with closed doors and windows	Yin and yang battle; yang extinguishes and yin abundant
Desires to climb high and sing, remove clothes and walk	Yin and yang battle again and combines with yang externally
Headache 頭痛 (tóu tòng) *Nasal Congestion* 鼻鼽 (bí qiú) *Abdominal Swelling* 腹腫 (fù zhǒng)	Yangming combines above with its tiny collaterals which belong to Taiyin

Taiyin conditions mentioned in Chapter 49

Distension 脹 (zhàng)	In the ninth month all things hide in the middle [jiāo]
Goes up to Heart 上走心 (shàng zǒu xīn) Leading to *Hiccups* 噫 (yī)	Yin abundant and goes up to the Yangming, which networks Heart
Postprandial Retching 食則嘔 (shí zé ǒu)	Substance abundant and full, overflows upward
Feel Good After Passing Stools or Gas 得後與氣則快然 (dé hòu yǔ qì zé kuài rán) *Frailty* 衰 (shuāi)	In the 12th month yin qi is frail, yang qi exits

Shaoyin conditions mentioned in Chapter 49

Low Back Pain 腰痛 (yāo tòng)	In the tenth month the yang qi of all things is harmed
Retching Cough (ǒu ké) 嘔欬 *Hyperventilation* 上氣 (shàng qì) *Panting* 喘 (chuǎn)	Yin qi below, yang qi above, all yang qi floats without anchor
Inability to Stand for Long Periods 色色不能久立 (sè sè bù néng jiǔ lì) *Vision blacks out when standing up after sitting too long, i.e. benign positional vertigo* 久坐起則目䀮䀮無所見 (jiǔ zuò qǐ zé mù máng máng wú suǒ jiàn)	Yin and yang of all things are not fixed, autumn qi arrives with slight frost to kill everything, yin and yang are robbed internally
Scant Qi 少氣 (shǎo qì) *Tendency to Anger* 善怒 (shàn nù)	Yang qi is not controlled and does not get to exit, Liver qi uncontrolled[116]
Fearful as if about to be arrested, i.e. paranoid 恐如人將捕之 (kǒng rú rén jiāng bǔ zhī)	In autumn, yin qi scant, yang qi enters, yin and yang battle

Averse to the Smell of Food 惡聞食臭 (wù wén shí chòu)	Stomach has no qi
Face Black as Ground 面黑如地色 (miàn hēi rú dì sè)	Autumn qi robs internally, therefore complexion changes
Cough leading to *Hemoptysis* or *Nosebleed*[117]	Yang vessels harmed, vessels full before yang qi abundant above, therefore see *Cough* and *Nosebleed*

Jueyin conditions mentioned in Chapter 49

Genital Hernia (tuí shàn) 癩疝 *Gynecological Hypogastric Swelling* 婦人少腹腫 (fù rén shào fù zhǒng)	In the third month the yin within yang is in the middle [jiāo]
Low Back and Spine Pain 腰脊痛 (yāo jǐ tòng) *Inability to Flex or Extend* 不可以俛仰 (bù kě yě fǔ yǎng)	In the third month when all is aroused[118]
Urine Retentive Genital Hernia (tuí lóng shàn) 癩癃疝 *Surface Distension* 膚脹 (fū zhàng)	Yin is also abundant
In extreme cases: *Esophageal Dryness* 嗌乾 (yì gān) *Heat Stroke* 熱中 (rè zhòng)	Yin and yang battle and create heat

Discussion on Pricking Essentials

刺要論

(cì yào lùn)

Chapter 50, Discussion on Pricking Essentials, is about needling depth.

The Emperor says, "[I am] willing to hear about the essentials to needling."*

Qi Bo replies, "Diseases can float or sink. Pricking can be shallow or deep." He goes on to explain that if you mistakenly needle into deeper† or shallower‡ levels than the one you are aiming for, it damages the five Zang internally and creates serious problems.

---

*   「願聞刺要」 (yuàn wén cì yào).

†   Pricking deeper than intended creates internal damage.

‡   Pricking shallower than intended creates external congestion, which creates susceptibility to external pathogens.

Needling depths and consequences

Disease location	Do not damage	Otherwise it affects / And causes
Fine hairs/ interstices	Skin	Lung
		溫瘧 (wēn nuè) *Warm Ague* 寒慄 (hán lì) *Cold Shivers* in autumn
Skin	Flesh	Spleen
		腹脹 (fù zhàng) *Abdominal Distension* 煩 (fán) *Vexation* 不嗜食 (bú shì shí) *Low Appetite* in between seasons[119]
Flesh	Vessel	Heart
		心痛 (xīn tòng) *Heart Pain*, i.e. angina, in summer
Vessel	Sinew	Liver
		熱 (rè) *Heat* 筋弛 (jīn chí) *Sinew Laxity* in spring
Sinew	Bone	Kidney
		脹 (zhàng) *Distension* 腰痛 (yāo tòng) *Low Back Pain* in winter
Bone	Marrow	N/A
		Emaciation 銷鑠 (xiāo shuò) *Shin Soreness* 脛酸 (jìng suān) *Lassitude* 解㑊 (xiè yì)

Discussion on Pricking Evenly

刺齊論

(cì qí lùn)

Chapter 51, Discussion on Pricking Evenly, is basically a how-to manual for the previous chapter.

The Emperor asks, "[I am] willing to hear about the difference in needling depths."

Qi Bo answers, "When needling bone, do not harm the sinew. When needling sinew, do not harm the flesh. When needling flesh, do not harm the vessel. When needling vessel, do not harm the skin. When needling skin, do not harm the flesh. When needling flesh, do not harm the sinew. When needling sinew, do not harm the bone."

Needling techniques for Chapter 50

To needle	Without harming	Technique
Bone	Sinew	Needle to sinew and remove, do not touch the bone
Sinew	Flesh	Needle to flesh and remove, do not touch the sinew
Flesh	Vessel	Needle to vessel and remove, do not touch the flesh
Vessel	Skin	Needle to skin and remove, do not touch the vessel
Skin	Flesh	Disease is in skin, so needle the skin
Flesh	Sinew	[Needle] past the flesh to touch the sinew
Sinew	Bone	[Needle] past the sinew to touch the bone

Discussion on Pricking Taboos

刺禁論

(cì jìn lùn)

Chapter 52, Discussion on Pricking Taboos, is about all the contraindications of acupuncture and their various consequences.

The (yào hài) 要害 "key vulnerabilities" of the Zang

肝生於左, 肺藏於右
(gān shēng yú zuǒ, fèi cáng yú yòu)
Liver generates from the left. Lung stores on the right.

心部於表, 腎治於裡
(xīn bù yú biǎo, shèn zhì yú lǐ)
Heart commands the exterior. Kidney governs the interior.

脾為之使, 胃為之市
(pí wéi zhī shǐ, wèi wéi zhī shì)
Spleen is the envoy. Stomach is the market.

隔肓之上, 中有父母
(gé huāng zhī shàng, zhōng yǒu fù mǔ)
Above the diaphragmatic membrane, in the center are father and mother.

七節之傍, 中有小心
(qī jié zhī báng, zhōng yǒu xiǎo xīn)
Beside the seven nodes, in the center is small heart.

從之有福, 逆之有咎
(cóng zhī yǒu fú, nì zhī yǒu jiù)
Following this there is prosperity. Countering this there is disaster.

Consequences of piercing organs during needling

Needle	Die in	Movement
Heart	1 day	*Burping* 噫 (yī)
Liver	5 days	*Raving* 語 (yǔ)
Kidney	6 days	*Sneezing* 嚏 (tì)
Lung	3 days	*Coughing* 欬 (ké)
Spleen	10 days	*Swallowing* 吞 (tūn)
Gallbladder	1.5 days	*Retching* 嘔 (ǒu)

Then the chapter goes into specific anatomical regions and contraindications against needling. Example: if the needle enters the brain via Du17*, instant death ensues. This part is a bit more difficult to understand.

---

*   腦戶 (nǎo hù) "Brain Window"

Cautions, contraindications and consequences of needling

Anatomical region	If needle	Consequence
Dorsum	Hits artery, bleeds nonstop	Death
Face	Hits blood vessel	Blindness
Du17[120]	Enters brain	Instant death
Sublingual vein	Too deep, bleeds nonstop	*Aphonia*
Under foot collateral vessel	No blood comes out	*Swelling*
Large popliteal vessel		*Syncope*[121] *Blanch*[122]
St30[123]	No blood comes out	*Inguinal Swelling*
Between vertebrae	Hits marrow	*Kyphosis*[124]
Breast	Hits breast	*Swelling* *Corrosion*[125]
Supraclavicular fossa[126]	Pneumothorax	*Cough* *Panting*
Hand thenar eminences[129]	Inserts into sunken area	*Swelling*

Here Qi Bo inserts a list of taboos, "Do not needle great intoxication, lest the qi become chaotic. Do not needle great wrath, lest the qi counterflow. Do not needle great depletion, nor those who have recently eaten, nor those who are greatly hungry, greatly thirsty, or greatly shocked." Then he returns to the list of contraindications and consequences.

Anatomical region	If needle	Consequence
Femoral artery	Causes nonstop bleeding	Death
GB3[128]	Causes internal leaking	*Deafness*
Patella	Causes fluids to extrude	*Lameness*
Arm Taiyin	Causes excessive bleeding	Instant death
Foot Shaoyin	Causes bleeding in very deficient patient	*Aphasia* (tongue difficult to talk)

Anatomical region	If needle	Consequence
Chest	Hits lung	*Panting* *Counterflow* *Supine Dyspnea**
Elbow	Causes qi to return	No flexion or extension
3 cùn below femoral groove		*Incontinence*
Armpit and intercostals		*Cough*
Hypogastrium	Hits bladder	*Urinary Incontinence* *Hypogastric Fullness*
UB56		*Swelling*
Eye socket	Hits vessel	*Leaking* *Blindness*
Joints	Fluid comes out	No flexion or extension

---

* 仰息 (yǎng xī) "supine audible exhalation"

Discussion on Pricking Recorded

刺志論

(cì zhì lùn)

Chapter 53, Discussion on Pricking Recorded, has nothing to do with the (zhì) 志 "willpower" involved with the five emotions. Instead the Emperor asks Qi Bo to elaborate on deficiency and excess. They go through common presentations, uncommon presentations, plus some basic definitions and techniques.

Uncommon presentations and their etiology

Presentation	Etiology
Qi abundant, body cold	傷寒 (shāng hán) *Cold Damage*
Qi deficient, body hot	傷暑 (shāng shǔ) *Summerheat Damage*
Eat a lot, but qi scanty	Losing blood and/or living in damp low places
Eat little, but qi copious	External pathogens in Stomach and Lung

Pulse small, but blood copious	飲 (yǐn) *Rheum* and 中熱 (zhōng rè) *Middle [jiāo] Heat*
Pulse big, but blood scanty	Vessel has wind qi blocking [the absorption of] food and water

Definitions of (shí) 實 and (xū) 虛 which I find valuable for understanding eight principles

實 (shí)	Qi enters	Hot	Open needle hole with left (supporting) hand
虛 (xū)	Qi exits	Cold	Close needle hole with left (supporting) hand

Chapters 50–53 are all pretty short. Clearly, length was not a consideration in the creation of this text. I think Chapter 5 is longer than all these chapters added up.

Needling Explanation

鍼解

(zhēn jiě)

Chapter 54, Needling Explanation, is again a chapter that supports the previous chapter's concepts with practical techniques. It explicates the proper approach to needling first mentioned in Chapter 25.

Needling techniques for insertion, removal, and retention

On insertion:
- When tonifying deficiency, the needle should feel hot
- When draining fullness, the needle should feel cold
- When eliminating stuff that has been accumulating over time, bad blood comes out

On removal:
- When there are external pathogens, do not close the hole
- To tonify, remove needle slowly and quickly close the hole
- To disperse, remove needle quickly and slowly close the hole

On retention:
- When pricking excess to create (xū) 虛 "space," retain the needle until yin qi arrives
- When pricking deficiency to create (shí) 實 "solidness," retain until yang qi arrives and the needle feels hot

Excess/Solidness (shí) 實 and deficiency/space (xū) 虛 are determined by the amount of cold and warm qi. If the disease does not appear to have a temperature, ask about chronology. When results are variable, the work has lost its principle. Align the time of tonification and dispersion with the opening and closing of qi.

Careful observation prevents mishaps and changes. The depth is in the willpower [of the practitioner] who knows whether the condition is internal or external. Distal and local are as one to [the practitioner who] waits at [the correct] depth. "As if before an abyss" means not daring to slack off. "As if holding a tiger" means with purpose and strength. Let the spirit be not concerned with the multitude things; quiet the mind and observe the patient without looking to the right or left.[*]

Point location of St36, St37, St39

That which is known as "Three Miles" (sān lǐ) 三里[†] is 3 cùn below the knee. That which is known as "Giant Mound" (jù xū) 巨虛[‡] is the indentation on the tibia when dorsiflexing the foot. That which is known as "Lower Ridge" (xià lián) 下廉[§] is a lower indentation.

I think the last paragraph is missing content because it doesn't make any sense. It reads like gobbledy-gook, but I doubt even the goblins from Harry Potter would be able to decipher it! I think it must have been miscopied, or otherwise damaged beyond reconstruction. I am encouraged that the *rest* of this book appears to make sense by comparison. Most editions of this chapter have **no punctuation** in the last paragraph. Although I have been using the Chinese Text Project[¶], and its characters/

---

[*]   I have omitted here 2–3 sentences about how to make the qi flow easily.

[†]   **Acu Trivia!** 三里 (sān lǐ): St36, known today as (zú sān lǐ) 足三里.

[‡]   **Acu Trivia!** 巨虛 (jù xū): St37, known today as (shàng jù xū) 上巨虛.

[§]   **Acu Trivia!** 下廉 (xià lián): St39, known today as (xià jù xū) 下巨虛. LI8 is known today as (xià lián) 下廉.

[¶]   https://ctext.org/huangdi-neijing/suwen

punctuation are none too accurate, usually it at least gives me hints as to where I might pause to draw breath.

Wang Bing agrees that the passage is corrupted and its meaning cannot be gleaned from what there is.

Discussion on Extended Pricking Guidelines

長刺節論

(cháng cì jié lùn)

Chapter 55, Discussion on Extended* Pricking Guidelines, seems to be on broad concepts of pricking various ailments, many of which have been mentioned in previous chapters. It also foregoes the question-and-answer format and is a straight lecture.

I like this quote at the beginning of the first paragraph:

刺家不診,
(cì jiā bù zhěn,)
Acupuncturists do not diagnose [based solely on observations],

聽病者言。
(tīng bìng zhě yán.)
[they] listen to the patient's words.

---

* This can mean extended needle retention or extended treatment through repeated techniques.

Needling techniques for various conditions

Disease	Technique
Headache 頭痛 (toú tòng)	Needle deeply to the bone without harming bone, flesh or skin
Cold Heat 寒熱 (hán rè)	陽刺 (yáng cì): insert 1 and 4 surrounding. Needle big Zang, if Zang is (pò) 迫[167] needle back-shū and Lv13 until the cold and heat subside. Slight bleeding during removal is essential
Rot Swelling 腐腫 (fǔ zhǒng)	Needle on the root according to size and depth of ulcer. Big ones will bleed a lot. For small ones, needle deeply and perpendicularly
Lower Abdominal Accumulation 少腹有積 (shào fù yǒu jī)	Needle locally perpendicularly, then add [Huà Tuó] Jiá Jǐ 華佗夾脊 at T4, GB29, and intercostal points bilaterally to descend heat in the abdomen
Hernia 疝 (shàn) abdominal pain, constipation/urine retention	Needle inner thighs, low back and hip points copiously until hypogastrium feels warm
Sinew Impediment 筋痹 (jīn bì) cramps, joint pain, and inability to walk	Needle on the sinew between the flesh[130] until sinew warms
Muscle Impediment 肌痹 (jī bì) myalgia all over from cold damp	Needle at origin and insertion of muscles copiously and deeply until muscles warm[131]
Bone Impediment 骨痹 (gǔ bì) due to cold qi with bone and marrow soreness, a sensation of heaviness with inability to lift bone	Needle deeply without harming vessel or flesh at origin and insertion until bones warm
Mania 狂 (kuáng) Disease in all yang vessels with alternating cold and heat	Needle deficient vessels until all [yang vessels] warm
Epilepsy[132] 癲病 (diān bìng)	Needle all the origins and insertions and all the vessels if there are no cold signs
Wind 風 (fēng) with alternating cold and heat and sweating multiple times a day	Needle collaterals of (fēn lǐ) 分理 muscle interstices and (còu lǐ) 腠理 interstices; if condition does not resolve immediately, treat once every 3 days for 100 days
Great Wind 大風 (dà fēng) with bone/joint heaviness and loss of eyebrows and sideburns	Needle muscle to induce sweating for 100 days, then needle bone and marrow to induce sweating for 100 days for a total of 200 days, until the eyebrows begin to grow back

Discussion on Skin Area

皮部論

(pí bù lùn)

Chapter 56 is called Discussion on Skin Areas, so I thought it would go into dermatology, but it does not. Mostly it covers collaterals and their pathological colors.

The Emperor says, "I have heard that the skin has (fēn bù) 分部 'designated areas,' the vessels have (jīng jì) 經紀 'channels and records,' the sinews have (jié luò) 節絡 'nodes [and] collaterals,' the bones have (dù liáng) 度量 'degrees [and] measurement,' which each have different diseases... I would like to hear about this."

Qi Bo answers, "The skin takes its discipline from the channels and vessels. All the vessels are thus. Yang of Yangming is called (hài fēi) 害蜚 *Harmful Cockroach*,* the varicosities in this area are all Yangming collaterals. If the color is green then pain, more black then (bì) 痹 *Impediment*, yellow and red are heat,

---

* 害蜚 (hài fēi): literally "harm cockroach!" Most historians say the characters are standing in for 闔 (hé) "Door-leaf" and 飛 (fēi) "Flight/Soar." I am not sure what that means either.

white is cold. If all five colors are present, then it is (hán rè) 寒熱 *Cold Heat*. If the collaterals are full then it lodges in the channels proper. Yang governs the outside. Yin governs the inside."

I have put the rest into a table for ease of reference. They pretty much all follow the description of *Harmful Cockroach*, except for the ones with additional notes.

Section	Name	Notes
Yang of Shaoyang	Pivot-holder 樞持 (shū chí)	At yang governs inside, at yin governs exit and seeps inward
Yang of Taiyang	Gate Pivot 關樞 (guān shū)	
Yin of Shaoyin	Pivot Scholar 樞儒 (shū rú)	Enters channels from yang area, enters bone from inside yin
Yin of Xīnzhǔ ("Heart Master", i.e. Pericardium)	Harm Shoulder 害肩 (hài jiān)	
Yin of Taiyin	Gate of Hibernating Insects 關蟄 (guān zhé)	

Discussion on Channels and Collaterals

經絡論

(jīng luò lùn)

Chapter 57, Discussion on Channels and Collaterals, wins the award for shortest chapter ever. It is about the colors of the (jīng) 經 "channels/meridians" versus the (luò) 絡 "collaterals/network vessels." Channels have a normal color; collaterals do not and change [colors] frequently. The channels and yin collaterals correspond to the five elements (Heart red, Lung white, Liver green, Spleen yellow, Kidney black); the yang collaterals change with the seasons (green and black when it is cold outside, yellow and red when it is hot). If all five colors are seen simultaneously, that indicates (hán rè) 寒熱 *Cold Heat*, i.e. a mixture of *Cold* and *Heat*.

Discussion on Qi Caves

氣穴論

(qì xué lùn)

Chapter 58, Discussion on Qi Caves,* must be an important chapter, because they go through the courtesies of the Golden Cabinet again, where Qi Bo demurs and the Emperor insists politely, promising that he will place this knowledge in the Golden Cabinet and not take it out again. So Qi Bo kowtows again and says, "For upper back and heart pain, treat R22, the tenth vertebra (Du7? The explanation makes it look like UB19) and R12.† The Zang have 50 shū-points. The Fu have 72 shū-points. Heat has 59 shū-points. Water has 57 shū-points. On the head there are five rows of five each, 25 acupoints. Along the

---

* Most of the time, when I see (xué) 穴 "cave" or (shū) 俞 "canoe" I translate it as "acupoint" (versus "point" which would be (diǎn) 點 in Chinese). The mental image conjured by these characters is so much more than an abstract dot. Most points do feel like caves to me on palpation, except the really congested ones, which feel as if they have been stopped up with stones.

† Qi Bo clarifies: 「(shàng jì) 上紀 "Upper Record" = R12, (xià jì) 下紀 "Lower Record" = R4」.

spine* there are five each, ten acupoints. Beside C7 there are two acupoints, one on each side. Speaking of two acupoints, there are:

2 near the eyes 浮白 (fú bái) "Floating White"	GB10 浮白 (fú bái)
2 in the hip socket	GB30 環跳 (huán tiào)
2 called 犢鼻 (dú bí) "Baby Ox Nose"	St35 犢鼻 (dú bí)
2 in the ears that help with hearing	SI19 聽宮 (tīng gōng)
2 at the root of the eyebrows	UB2 攢竹 (zǎn zhú)
2 at 完骨 (wán guˇ) the "mastoid process"	GB12 完骨 (wán gǔ)
1 at the center of the nape	Du16 風府 (fēng fǔ)
2 on the occipital bone	GB20 風池 (fēng chí)
2 "above the jaw" 上關 (shàng guān)	GB3 上關 (shàng guān)
2 "below the jaw" 下關 (xià guān)	St7 下關 (xià guān)
2 called 天柱 (tiān zhù) "Sky Pillar"	UB10 天柱 (tiān zhù)
4 above and below (jù xū) 巨虛 the "giant void"	St37 上巨虛 (shàng jù xū) St39 下巨虛 (xià jù xū)
2 at the bend of the teeth	St6 頰車 (jiá chē)
1 called 天突 (tiān tú) "Sky Protrusion"	R22 天突 (tiān tú)
2 called 天府 (tiān fǔ) "Sky Mansion"	Lu3 天府 (tiān fǔ)
2 called 天牖 (tiān yǒu) "Sky Wall-window"	SJ16 天牖 (tiān yǒu)
2 called 扶突 (fú tú) "Support Protrusion"	LI18 扶突 (fú tú)
2 called 天窗 (tiān chuāng) "Sky Window"[133]	SI16 天窗 (tiān chuāng)
2 for "Shoulder Release" 肩解 (jiān jiě)	GB21 肩井 (jiān jǐng)
1 called 關元 (guān yuán) "Gate Origin"	R4 關元 (guān yuán)
2 called 委陽 (wěi yáng) "Bend Yang"	UB39 委陽 (wěi yáng)
2 called 肩貞 (jiān zhēn) "Shoulder True"	SI9 肩貞 (jiān zhēn)
1 called 瘖門 (yīn mén) "Aphonic Door"	Du15 啞門 (yǎ mén)
1 at the navel	R8 神闕 (shén què)

---

* Here is another character my computer cannot type…the flesh radical 月 next to 呂 which is pronounced (lǚ)…it means "backbone," and I am pronouncing it based on the right side, hoping it is a phono-semantic character.

12 shū-points on the chest	K22–27
2 shū-points on the back	UB11 大杼 (dà zhù)
12 shū-points on the lateral chest[134]	Lu1–2, Sp19–21
2 points called 分肉 (fēn ròu) "Divide Flesh"	GB38 陽輔 (yáng fǔ)
2 points above the ankle	K9 交信 (jiāo xìn)
4 points of the yin/yang qiao	K6 照海 (zhào hǎi) UB62 申脈 (shēn mài)

The water-shū points are at all the divisions. The heat-shū points are at qi caves. *Cold Heat* shū-points are the two points GB33. [There are] 25 great taboos. 5 cùn below Lu3.* All 365 acupoints may be moved by needling."

The Emperor then asks about collateral vessels and Qi Bo answers, "There are 365 meeting caves here to reflect one year too. If qi and blood are depleted, it will (fā rè) 發熱 *Express Heat* externally, [and manifest as] (shǎo qì) 少氣 *Scant Qi* internally."

The Emperor says, "[I] am willing to hear of the meeting of streams and valleys."

Qi Bo answers, "The great meetings of flesh are valleys, the small meetings of flesh are streams. Between the flesh, streams and valleys move the defensive and nutritive qi to meet large qi. When external pathogens overflow, qi is congested, vessels heat up, flesh is defeated, defensive and nutritive qi do not move; the result is pus in the bone and marrow. If cold accumulates, the muscles contract and sinews shrink, extension becomes impossible. This great cold lingering in streams and valleys creates (gǔ bì) 骨痹 *Bone Impediment* internally and (bù rén) 不仁 *Numbness* externally. The streams and valleys meet at 365 caves, also reflecting one year. Small impediments and overflows may be treated similarly."

The Emperor is very excited by this information and reiterates that he will store it in the (jīn guì) 金匱 "Golden Cabinet" of his (jīn lán zhī shì) 金蘭之室 "Golden Lotus Room."

---

* I suspect we might be missing half a sentence here.

Qi Bo adds that the (sūn luò) 孫絡 "grandchildren collaterals," i.e. the capillaries, should be drained when full, and that there are 365 of those that flow into the 12 luò-collaterals. I am not quite sure of the significance of this long list of points yet, but I am putting it in the Golden Cabinet of my mind and coming back to it in time.

Discussion on Qi Mansions

氣府論

(qì fǔ lùn)

Chapter 59, Discussion on Qi Mansions, consists of a long list of acupoints "where the vessel qi expresses" from the following channels, with anatomical positions rather than names (except the acupoints whose names are anatomical). I am putting modern point numbers for easier reference, with unexpected points and locations in *italics*.

Foot Taiyang 78 acupoints

2 on eyebrows	UB2
3.5 cùn from hairline toward the crown	*Du22, Du23, Du24*
25 (5×5) floating qi in middle of scalp	5 lines of 5 points from Prefrontal 5[135]
2 beside the big occipital sinew	UB10
2 beside (fēng fǔ) 風府 Du16	*GB20*
Along back to the sacrum on either side of the 21 joints and 15 vertebral spaces	UB41–UB54 and UB36

5 back-shū points for each of the 5 Zang	UB13, UB15, UB18, UB20, UB23
6 back-shū points for each of the 6 Fu	UB19, UB21, UB22, UB25, UB27, UB28
6 shū-points from UB40 down to the lateral edge of the little toe	UB40, UB60, UB64, UB65, UB66, UB67

Foot Shaoyang 62 acupoints

2 above the corner [of the head]	GB7, GB9
Above pupil up into the hairline 5 each	GB15, GB16, GB17, GB18, GB19
1 each above the front corner of the ear	GB4
1 each below the front corner of the ear	GB5
1 each below the sideburns	*SJ22*
1 each called (kè zhǔ rén) 客主人	GB3
1 each in the hollow behind the ear	*SJ17*
1 each lower mandible	*St7*
1 each behind the lower teeth below the ear	*St6*
1 each in the supraclavicular fossa	*St12*
8 from 3 cùn in the intercostals 3 cùn below the ribs to hypochondria	GB22, GB23, GB24, GB26, GB27, GB29, *P1, Lv13*
1 each in the hip socket	GB30
6 each from knee to fourth little toe	GB34, GB38, GB40, GB41, GB43, GB44

Foot Yangming 68 acupoints

3 each in hairline along forehead	St8, *GB5, GB14*
1 each in the hollow of the facial bone	St2
2 each in the hollow of the jawbone	St5
1 each at (rén yíng) 人迎	St9
1 each in the hollow of the bone lateral to (quē pén) 缺盆 St12	*SJ15*
1 each in the central bone of the lateral chest	St13, St14, St15, St17, St18
5 each along (jiū wěi) 鸠尾 Ren15 *3 cùn* below the breast and along the epigastrium	St19, St20, St21, St22, St23

3 each along the navel *3 cùn wide*	St24, St25, St26
3 each below the navel 2 cùn wide	St27, St28, St29
1 each in the artery at (qì jiē) 氣街	St30
1 each above (fú tù) 伏兔	St31
8 each from (sān lǐ) 三里 St36 to the *middle toe* of the foot	St36, St37, St39, St41, St42, St43, St44, St45

Hand Taiyang 36 acupoints

1 each inner eye canthus	*UB1*
1 each outer eye [canthus]	*GB1*
1 each below the cheekbone[136]	SI18
1 each above auricle	*SJ20*
1 each in center of ear	SI19
1 each at (jù gǔ) 巨骨 the "acromioclavicular joint"?	*LI15*
1 each above armpit crease in a foramen	SI9
1 each in the indentation on the clavicle	*GB21*
1 each *4 cùn above (tiān chuāng)* 天窗 *SI16*	*GB11*
1 each for (jiān jiě) 肩解 "Shoulder Relief"	SI12
1 each 3 cùn below Shoulder Relief	SI11
6 each from elbow to pinky finger	SI8, SI5, SI4, SI3, SI2, SI1

Hand Yangming 22 acupoints

2 each lateral to the nostrils	LI20, LI19?
1 each in the hollow of the jawbone named (dà yíng) 大迎 St5	LI18
1 each where clavicular bone meets	LI17
1 each where humerus meets	LI15
6 each from below the elbow to the root of thumb and forefinger	LI10, LI5, LI4, LI3, LI2, LI1

Hand Shaoyang 32 acupoints

1 each below the nasal congestion bone	*SI18*
1 each behind the eyebrow	SJ23
1 each above the corner [of the head]	*GB4*
1 each below and behind (wán gǔ) 完骨 GB12	SJ16
1 each in the nape anterior to Foot Taiyang	*GB20*
1 each along LI18	*SI16*
1 each at (jiān zhēn) 肩貞	*SI9*
1 each in the space 3 cùn below (jiān zhēn) 肩貞	SJ12, SJ13, SJ14
6 each from below the elbow to ring finger	SJ10, SJ6, SJ4, SJ3, SJ2, SJ1

Dū-Governing 28 acupoints

2 in center of nape	Du15, Du16
8 in posterior hairline	Du17–24
3 in center of face	Du25, Du26, Du27
15 beside from C7 to sacrum	Du1–14, *UB35*

There are 21 [vertebral] joints from C7 to the coccyx.

Rèn-Controlling 28 acupoints

2 in center of throat	Ren22, Ren23
1 each in indentation of sternum	Ren17, Ren18, Ren19, Ren20, Ren21
1 3 cùn below (jiū wěi) 鳩尾 Ren15	Ren14, Ren15
5 cùn to (zhōng wǎn) 中脘 Ren12	Ren9–13
6.5 cùn from navel to pubic symphysis	Ren2–7
1 at perineum	Ren1
1 each below the eyes	??
1 at the lower lip	Ren24
1 at (yín jiāo) 齦交 the gumline	*Du28*

Chōng-penetrating 22 acupoints

1 each every 0.5 cùn [along Ren] 0.5 cùn from (jiū wěi) 鳩尾 R15	*K17–K21*
1 each every 0.5 cùn from navel to pubic symphysis	*K11–K16*

Additional points mentioned in Chapter 59

Foot Shaoyin has 1 below the tongue	*Ren23*
[Foot] Jueyin has 1 at the border of the pubic hair	Lv12
Hand Shaoyin has 1	H6
Yin/Yang Qiao have 1 each	K6/UB62
The thenar eminences of the hands and feet are also points	Lu10, K1?

Vessel qi expresses at the (yú jì) 魚際 "fish borders" of the hands and feet* through these 365 acupoints.

---

*   I think this means the thenar eminence, hypothenar eminence, and maybe the abductor hallucis and the abductor digiti minimi. **Acu Trivia!** (yú jì) 魚際 is the name of Lu10.

Chapter 60

Discussion on Bone Spaces

骨空論

(gǔ kōng lùn)

Chapter 60, Discussion on Bone Spaces, is a juicy chapter with more on treating (fēng) 風 *Wind* with acupuncture, acupoint locations, pathological conditions for the Ren, Du, the knee joint, the 57 water-shū points (I have never heard of this, and the previous chapter did not explain), the bone spaces that the chapter is named for, and how to moxa (hán rè) 寒熱 *Cold Heat*.

The Emperor starts by asking, "I have heard that wind is the beginning of a hundred diseases. How do [you] treat it with needles?"

Qi Bo answers, "When wind enters from without, creating chills, sweating, headache, a sensation of heaviness in the body and aversion to cold, treat with (fēng fǔ) 風府 'wind mansion' Du16, regulate the yin and yang, tonify deficiency, drain excess."

Wind-related signs and symptoms mentioned in Chapter 60

Sign/symptom	Treatment
Big Wind 大風 (dà fēng) *Neck/Nape Pain* 頸項痛 (jǐng xiàng tòng)	Needle (fēng fǔ) 風府 "Wind Mansion" Du16
Big Wind 大風 (dà fēng) *Sweating* 汗出 (hàn chū)	Moxa āshì point(s) 3 cùn lateral to [Huà Tuó] Jiá Jǐ āshì points
Abhorrence of Wind 憎風 (zēng fēng)	Needle eyebrow
Losing Pillow 失枕 (shī zhěn) acute torticollis	Moxa (jǐ zhōng) 脊中 "Spine Center" Du6
Pain/Distension 痛脹 (tòng zhàng) from floating ribs radiating to hypogastrium	Needle āshì
Low Back Pain 腰痛 (yāo tòng) with *Inability to Laterally Rotate* 不可以轉搖 (bù kě yǐ zhuǎn yáo)	Needle 八髎 (bā liáo) "8 foramen" UB31–34 and above the pain
Mouse Fistula 鼠瘻 (shǔ lòu) *Cold Heat* 寒熱 (hán rè)	Needle 寒府 (hán fǔ) "Cold Mansion" GB33 lateral bone seam of knee joint

任脈 (rèn mài) Controlling Vessel

Origin: under (zhōng jí) 中極 "Center Pole" R3

Follows pubic hair up (guān yuán) 關元 "Gate Origin" R4 to throat, up cheeks along the face into the eyes

Diseases:
Men:
Internal Knots 內結 (nèi jié)
Seven Hernias 七疝 (qī shàn)
Women:
Leukorrhea 帶下 (dài xià)
Conglomeration and Gatherings 瘕聚 (jiǎ jù)

沖脈 (chōng mài) Penetrating Vessel

Origin: (qì jiē) 氣街 "Qi Street" St30

Follows Shaoyin Channel up along navel to center of chest

Diseases:
Counterflow Qi 逆氣 (nì qì)
Tenesmus 裡急 (lǐ jí)

督脈 (dū mài) Governing Vessel

Origin: center of bone below hypogastrium (women: connected to urethral opening)

Networks and circles genitals and buttocks to Shaoyin, joins the Juyang, goes through the spine to inner canthus, forehead, crown, networks brain, branches out nape to shoulders, goes inward down the spine (men: follows penis to (cuàn) 篡 "usurpation"? Wiseman translates this as perineum), travels center of navel up (yí) 頤 "cheek/jaw" to circle the lips

Diseases:
Spinal Stiffness 脊強 (jǐ jiàng)
Tonic Spasm 反折 (fǎn zhé)
Rushing Hernia[137] 沖疝 (chōng shàn)
Women only:
Infertility 不孕 (bú yùn)
Urinary Retention 癃 (lóng)
Hemorrhoids 痔 (zhì)
Enuresis 遺溺 (yí niào)
Esophageal Dryness 嗌乾 (yì gān)

Treatment: on the bone, or for extreme cases in area below navel, on the throat if there is audible breathing

Treating *Knee Pain*

If the knee extends and cannot flex treat the (jiàn) 楗 between fibula and pubic bones

If sitting causes knee pain treat the (jī) 機 the side of the hip

If standing and summer relieves, treat the (hái guān) 骸關 the knee joint

If knee pain radiates to the big toe, treat the (guó) 膕 the popliteal crease

If sitting creates knee pain and a sensation of hidden obstructions, treat the (guān) 關 above the popliteal crease

Knee pain with inability to flex or extend, treat the (bèi nèi) 背內 "Inner Spine" UB11

If the calves feel broken, treat the (zhōng shū liáo) 中俞髎 "center acupoint foramen" of Yangming, i.e. St36, St43, and/or St37[138]

If knees feel (bié) 別 "divergent" treat UB65 and K2

If calves are sore and cannot endure standing, treat the (wéi) 維 "linking" of Shaoyang 5 cùn up, i.e. GB38

On 57 water-shū points*

5 rows on the sacrum, 5 points per row
2 rows on (fú tù) 伏兔 "Crouching Rabbit" St32, 5 points per row
1 row each on right and left, 5 points per row
1 row each above ankle, 6 points per row

On moxa for (hán rè) 寒熱 *Cold Heat*

Begin with Du14, moxa the number of cones by [the patient's age in] years
Then moxa the coccyx (Du1), number of cones by year
Moxa the indented back-shū points
Raise the arm and moxa the indented points on top of the shoulder
Moxa between the ribs (GB25) bilaterally
Moxa the end of the fibula above the lateral malleolus (GB38)
Moxa between the fourth and fifth toes (GB44)
Moxa the indented vessel below the gastrocnemius (UB57)
Moxa behind the lateral malleolus (UB60)
Moxa the hard, painful sinewy area above St12
Moxa the lateral chest indentation between bones
Moxa beneath the metacarpal (P7 or SJ4)
Moxa 3 cùn below the navel (R4)
Moxa the artery at the edge of the pubic hair (R6)
Moxa 3 cùn below the knee (St36)
Moxa the Foot Yangming dorsal artery (St42)
Moxa 1 atop the head (Du20)
Moxa 3 cones at area of dog-bite in the method of treating dog-inflicted injuries
All these 29 spots ought to receive moxibustion

If treating (shāng shí) 傷食 *Food Damage* by moxa does not yield results, one must observe where the channel passes more yang, needle that shū-point multiple times, and then apply medicine.

---

*   After the section on water-shū points, I have omitted an anatomical paragraph.

Discussion on Water Heat Caves

水熱穴論

(shuǐ rè xué lùn)

Chapter 61, Discussion on Water Heat Caves, is about Kidney water and its relationship to Lung. More specifically, it is about Kidney Shaoyin's relationship to Lung Taiyin. It explicates and explains acupoint prescriptions for lymphedema and ascites, shortness of breath, the inability to lie supine. There are also explanations for seasonal pricking techniques that explain Dr. Tan's 12 Magic Points. Finally, it offers an explanation for *Heat* as arising from *Cold Damage*.

A key symptom of Kidney issues is (fú zhǒng) 胕腫 *Puffy Swelling*, i.e. edema. Qi Bo explains, "Kidney is the Gate of Stomach. If the Gate does not open and close smoothly, it gathers water pathologically creating *Puffy Swelling*." He goes on to explain that heroic exertion causes the Kidney to sweat, and if Kidney sweating occurs in conjunction with *Wind* that gets lodged in the pores, it will travel inside the skin to become *Puffy Swelling* that originates from the Kidney, also known as (fēng shuǐ) 風水 *Wind Water*.

Symptoms of *Water Disease* below (in the Kidney) are edema and enlarged abdomen; above (in the Lung) are panting [on] exhalation and inability to lie flat. The two rows of five acupoints each on (fú tù) 伏兔 "Crouching Rabbit" St32 on the thigh are the "streets of Kidney"; there are also the lower rows of Kidney called (tài chōng) 太沖 "Great Rushing," one row above each ankle of six acupoints each. Of the 57 acupoints, all are yin collaterals of the Zang where water lodges.

Seasonal pricking explanations

In spring, we needle the origins and insertions of muscles because Liver qi flows urgently and wind creates diseases, and there is not enough qi yet for deep pricking. In summer, we needle abundance shallowly because yang qi is overflowing from Heart qi growing and heat is smoking the flesh and interstices. In autumn, we choose jīng-river points because yin qi is returning to conquer yang but has not yet had a chance to go deep; we choose back-shū points to drain yin pathogens, and hé-sea points to empty yang pathogens as yang qi begins to decline. In winter, we choose jǐng-well points to lower yin counterflow and yíng-spring points to solidify yang qi. Dr Tan's *12 Magical Points* begins in winter and cycles through the seasons limb by limb.

59 acupoints for treating *Heat Disease*

Qi Bo says, "There are five rows of five on the head to clear heat counterflow of all yang. The eight acupoints (dà zhù) 大杼 'big loom-shuttle' UB11, (yīng shū) 膺俞 'lateral-chest shu' Lu1, (quē pén) 缺盆 'chipped basin' St12, (bèi shū) 背俞 'upper-back shu' UB12 drain heat from the chest. The eight acupoints (qì jiē) 氣街 'qi street' St30, (sān lǐ) 三里 'Three Miles'* St36,

---

* Actually, 1 lǐ 里 is a unit of distance that measures 500m or approximately one third of a mile, so technically (sān lǐ) 三里 is the distance of one mile.

巨虛上下廉 (jù xū shàng xià lián) 'upper and lower ridge [of] giant ruin' St37 and St39 drain heat from the Stomach. The eight acupoints (yú mén) 'cloud door' 雲門 Lu2, (yú gǔ) 髃骨 'clavicle bone' LI15, (wěi zhōng) 委中 'popliteal center' UB40, (suí kōng) 髓空 'marrow space' Du2 drain heat from the four limbs. The ten acupoints beside the back-shū of the Five Zang (unnamed in text, UB42, UB44, UB47, UB49, UB52) drain heat from the five Zang. All 59 of these acupoints are the left and right of *Heat*."

Cold Damage transforms to Heat

The Emperor asks one last question, "Why does *Cold Damage* transform into *Heat*?"

Qi Bo says, "When *Cold* is exuberant, it generates *Heat*." I believe this happens because cold constricts and obstructs the natural flow of qi, which is yang, i.e. warm in nature, because we are warm-blooded mammals, and when qi gets stuck in one place unable to flow, it turns into pathological heat. At least, this is one way excess cold may result in heat.

Discussion on Regulating Channels

調經論

(tiáo jīng lùn)

Chapter 62, Discussion on Regulating Channels, describes tonifying and draining needling techniques. The basic premise is to disperse where there is excess, and to tonify where there is deficiency. It also outlines components of eight principles diagnosis (deficiency/excess, yin/yang, cold/heat) in terms of a concept I have never seen before called (bìng) 并 "merge".

The chapter begins with the Emperor asking Qi Bo how the jīng-essence, qi, body fluids, four limbs, nine orifices, five Zang, 16 areas, and 365 joints can be reduced to five excesses and five deficiencies. Qi Bo answers, "[Deficiency and excess are] all generated by the five Zang." He goes on to explain:

Zang	Hides
Heart	Spirit
Lung	Qi
Liver	Blood
Spleen	Body
Kidney	Will

Treatments for (yǒu yú) 有餘 excess

	Excess symptoms	Treatment
Spirit	*Laugh Nonstop* 笑不休 (xiào bù xiū)	Drain blood from small collaterals
Qi	*Panting Cough* 喘欬 (chuǎn ké) *Hyperventilation* 上氣 (shàng qì)	Drain (jīng suì) 經隧 "channel tunnel" without releasing blood or qi
Blood	*Anger* 怒 (nù)	Bleed excess channels
Form	*Abdominal Distension* 腹脹 (fù zhàng) *Urinary Inhibition* 涇溲不利 (jīng sōu bú lì)	Drain yang channel
Willpower	*Abdominal Distension* 腹脹 (fù zhàng) *Lienteric Diarrhea* 飧泄 (sūn xiè)	Drain sinews and blood

Treatment for (bù zú) 不足 deficiency

	Symptoms	Treatment
Spirit	*Sadness* 悲 (bēi)	Massage/Needle deficient collaterals without letting out blood or qi
Qi	*Breathing Uninhibited* 息利 (xī lì) *Scant Qi* 少氣 (shǎo qì)	Tonify (jīng suì) 經隧 "channel tunnel" without letting qi out
Blood	*Fear* 恐 (kǒng)	Needle deficient channels at vessel depth, long retention, quick removal without letting blood drain
Form	*Four Limbs No Use* 四肢不用 (sì zhī bú yòng)	Tonify yang collateral
Willpower	*Reversal* 厥 (jué)	Tonify K7

The Emperor says, "Ah. Now I have heard the shape of (xū) 虛 and (shí) 實, but I do not know how they are generated." Qi Bo gives some examples of how qi and blood may (bìng) 并 "combine/merge" to create the following conditions.

Qi and blood (bìng) 并 merge

Condition	~ merges with ~
Shock Mania 驚狂 (jīng kuáng)	Blood merges with yin Qi merges with yang
Intense Heat [in] Middle 炅中 (jiǒng zhōng)	Blood merges with yang Qi merges with yin
Heart Vexation Regret 心煩惋 (xīn fán wǎn) *Tendency for Anger* 善怒 (shàn nù)	Blood merges with above Qi merges with below
Chaotic and Forgetful 亂而喜忘 (luàn ér xǐ wàng)	Blood merges with below Qi merges with above

Blood and qi like warmth and are averse to cold. Cold congeals flow. Warmth dissolves. Therefore qi creates *Blood Deficiency*; blood's bìng-merge creates qi deficiency. Qi Bo goes deeper into these concepts for a few eloquent and confusing sentences about the xū and shí of blood bìng versus qi bìng.

Qi Bo then categorizes external pathogens in terms of yin and yang. Wind, rain, cold, and heat (i.e. weather) create yang problems. Diet, living conditions, and emotions create yin problems. The term "exterior" (biǎo) 表 is not mentioned, but the "solid" 實 (shí) progression of disease through skin-capillaries-collaterals-channels and its effect on the nutritive and defensive qi describe exterior invasion pretty exactly. The "solid" 實 (shí) progression of yin qi counterflowing upward when we are angry creates "emptiness" 虛 (xū) below; qi dissipates when we are sad creating "emptiness" 虛 (xū) within the vessels.

Manifestations of deficiency versus excess

	Deficient 虛 (xū)	Exuberant 盛 (shèng)		Deficient 虛 (xū)	Exuberant 盛 (shèng)
Yang	External cold	External heat	Yin	Internal heat	Internal cold

The second to last paragraph reiterates key pricking techniques for draining (remove needle with wiggling motion to open a passageway and release qi) versus tonifying (awaiting the exhalation to insert needle, removing quickly, etc.).

The final question and answer explains how regulating the five Zang can treat excess and deficiency of the 12 channels and vessels and 365 joints.

Discussion on Contralateral-Collateral Pricking

繆刺論

(miù cì lùn)

Chapter 63, Discussion on Contralateral-Collateral Pricking, describes acupuncture for a variety of conditions, most of which affect the luò-collaterals.

The first paragraph clarifies the difference between (jù cì) 巨刺 "contralateral-channel pricking" which is done to the jīng-channels versus (miù cì) 繆刺 "contralateral-collateral' pricking which is done to the luò-collaterals to clear external pathogens.

Specific acupoint prescriptions for various conditions mentioned in Chapter 63

External pathogen in	Signs and symptoms	Treatment (if not immediately cured, add ~)
Foot Shaoyin luò	*Sudden Angina* 卒心痛 (cù xīn tòng) *Violent Distension* 暴脹 (bào zhàng) *Chest/Rib Propping Fullness* 胸脇支滿 (xiōng xié zhī mǎn) without [signs of] *Accumulation* 積 (jī)	Bleed K2, 5 days
Hand Shaoyang luò	*Throat Impediment* 喉痹 (hóu bì) *Aphasia* 舌卷 (shé juǎn) *Mouth Dryness* 口乾 (kǒu gān) *Heart Vexation* 心煩 (xīn fán) *Lateral Arm Pain* 臂外廉痛 (bì wài lián tòng) *Inability to Reach Head* 手不及頭 (shǒu bù jí tóu)	Bleed P9, SJ1
Foot Jueyin luò	*Sudden Hernia* 卒疝 (cù shàn) *Violent Pain* 暴痛 (bào tòng)	Bleed Lv1
Foot Taiyang luò	*Head/Nape/Shoulder Pain* 頭項肩痛 (tóu xiàng jiān tòng)	Bleed UB67, (UB62)
Hand Yangming luò	*Qi Fullness* 氣滿 (qì mǎn) *Chest/Center Panting* 胸中喘息 (xiōng zhōng chuǎn xī) *Armpit/Torso/Chest/Center Heat* 支胠胸中熱 (zhī qū xiōng zhōng rè)	Bleed Lu11, LI1
Between arm and hand	*Difficulty with Flexion* 不可得曲 (bù kě dé qū)	Needle trigger points
Foot Yang Qiao Vessel	*Eye Pain* 目痛 (mù tòng) starting at inner canthus	Bleed UB62

Blood Stasis from traumatic fall	*Abdominal/Central Fullness* 滿 (mǎn) and *Distension* 脹 (zhàng) with constipation and urine retention	Drink diuretics/laxatives, bleed K6, K2, St42, (R4??)
	Tendency for Sadness 善悲 (shàn bēi) *Shock* 驚 (jīng) *Lacking Joy* 不樂 (bú lè)	Same as above
Hand Yangming luò	*Deafness* 耳聾 (ěr lóng) occasional *Tinnitus* 耳中生風 (ěr zhōng shēng fēng)	Bleed Lu11, LI1, (P9)
All (bì) 痹 *Impediment* that moves around		Needle painful origins and insertions, number by birth month
Foot Yangming jīng -Channel	*Nosebleed* 鼽衄 (qiú nù) *Upper Teeth Cold* 上齒寒 (shàng chǐ hán)	Bleed St44 and middle toe
Foot Shaoyang luò	*Rib Pain* on exhalation 脇痛 (xié tòng) *Cough* 欬 (ké) with *Sweating* 汗出 (hàn chū)	Bleed UB67, GB44
Foot Shaoyin luò	*Esophageal Pain* with inability to ingest food 嗌痛 (yì tòng) *Tendency for Anger* 善怒 (shàn nù) and/or *Qi Ascension* for no reason 氣上 (qì shàng)	Needle K1
	Esophageal Swelling 嗌中腫 (yì zhōng zhǒng) with inability to ingest [food] or expel spittle	Needle K2

External pathogen in	Signs and symptoms	Treatment (if not immediately cured, add ~)
Foot Taiyin luò	*Low Back Pain* 腰痛 (yāo tòng) radiating to hypogastrium and floating ribs with inability to extend	Needle sacrum, number by birth month
Foot Taiyang luò	*Hypertonicity* 拘攣 (jǔ luán) in upper back radiating pain to ribs	Needle painful Jiá Jǐ
Foot Shaoyang luò	*Hip Pain with Inability to Lift Thigh* 樞中痛髀不可舉 (shū zhōng tòng bì bù kě jǔ)	Needle hip joint[139] number by birth month
	Deafness 耳聾 (ěr lóng)	Needle Hand Yangming (points anterior to ear canal)
	Tooth Decay 齒齲 (chǐ qǔ)	Needle Hand Yangming (vessels that enter the teeth)
Between five Zang	Vessels hurt on and off 脈引而痛，時來時止 (mài yǐn ér tòng, shí lái shí zhǐ)	Bleed nail (jǐng-well) points every other day for 5 days
	Teeth/Lips Cold Pain 齒脣寒痛 (chǐ chún hán tòng)	Bleed back of hand and P9, LI1, Lu11
Hand/Foot Shaoyin/ Taiyin Foot Yangming luò which meet inside the ear	*Corpse Reversal* 屍厥 (shī jué), i.e. body and vessels all move, yet form unconscious as a corpse	Bleed Lv1, then needle K1, middle toenail, Lu11, P7 and H7 in sequence

There are actually specifics about needle depth or bloodletting techniques for most of these treatments which are not included in the chart.

In conclusion, when needling, first look at and palpate the jīng-channels and mài-vessels to determine (xū) 虛 "deficiency" and (shí) 實 "excess". Needle the jīng-channels if they are disregulated. Use (miù cì) 繆刺 "contralateral-collateral pricking" if there is pain but the channels are not disregulated, and bleed the luò-collaterals wherever you see changes on the skin.

Discussion on Pricking Against or With the Flow of the Four Seasons

四時刺逆從論

(sì shí cì nì cóng lùn)

Chapter 64, Discussion on Pricking Against or With the Flow of the Four Seasons, lays out general causes for many types of *Impediment*, *Hernia*, and *Accumulation*, sketches the depth at which pathogens lodge within the body during each season, and details the consequences of inappropriate needle depth. It also reiterates five types of death caused by directly harming the five Zang through incorrect needling.

Etiology

	Jueyin	Shaoyin	Taiyin
Excess 有餘 (yǒu yú)	*Yin Impediment* 陰痹 (yīn bì)	*Skin Impediment* 皮痹 (pí bì)	*Flesh Impediment* 肉痹 (ròu bì)
Insufficient 不足 (bù zú)	*Heat Impediment* 熱痹 (rè bì)	*Lung Impediment* 肺痹 (fèi bì)	*Spleen Impediment* 脾痹 (pí bì)
Slippery 滑 (huá)	*Fox Hernia* 狐疝 (hú shàn)	*Lung Wind Hernia* 肺風疝 (fèi fēng shàn)	*Spleen Wind Hernia* 脾風疝 (pí fēng shàn)
Rough 澀 (sè)	*Accumulation of Qi* 積氣 (jī qì) in lower abdomen	*Accumulation Hematuria* 積溲血 (jī sōu xiě)	*Accumulation of Heart and Abdomen with Periodic Fullness* 積心腹時滿 (jī xīn fù shí mǎn)

	Yangming	Taiyang	Shaoyang
Excess 有餘 (yǒu yú)	*Vessel Impediment* 脈痹 (mài bì) with periodic hot flashes	*Bone Impediment* 骨痹 (gǔ bì) with body heaviness	*Sinew Impediment* 筋痹 (jīn bì) with 脇滿 (xié mǎn) *Rib Fullness*
Insufficient 不足 (bù zú)	*Heart Impediment* 心痹 (xīn bì)	*Kidney Impediment* 腎痹 (shèn bì)	*Liver Impediment* 肝痹 (gān bì)
Slippery 滑 (huá)	*Heart Wind Hernia* 心風疝 (xīn fēng shàn)	*Kidney Wind Hernia* 腎風疝 (shèn fēng shàn)	*Liver Wind Hernia* 肝風疝 (gān fēng shàn)
Rough 澀 (sè)	*Accumulation with Periodic Shock* 積時善驚 (jī shí shàn jīng)	*Accumulation with Periodic Vertex Disease* 積善時巔疾 (jī shàn shí diān jí)	*Accumulation with Periodic Sinew Cramps and Eye Pain* 積時筋急目痛 (jī shí jīn jí mù tòng)

Where the qi resides in which season, and why

	Qi at	Explanation[140]
Spring	Channels/Vessels 經脈 (jīng mài)	Sky qi begins to open, land qi begins to drain, ice melts to water and begins to flow
Summer	Capillaries/Collaterals 孫絡 (sūn luò)	Channels fill and qi overflows into capillaries and collaterals, making skin and surface "solidifies" 實 (shí)
Longsummer	Muscles/Flesh 肌肉 (jī ròu)	Both channels and collaterals are abundant, overflowing into the muscles
Autumn	Skin/Surface 皮膚 (pí fū)	Sky qi begins to collect, interstices close up, the skin and surface tighten
Winter	Bone/Marrow 骨髓 (gǔ suí)	Hibernation (cover[141] and hide[142]), blood and qi pour into bones and marrow, connect to the five Zang

"Thus pathogens follow the qi and blood of the four seasons to lodge within. Though they may ultimately change and transform in immeasurable ways, they must follow the qi of the channels. If the pathogen is dispelled, chaotic qi cannot be generated."

The Emperor asks, sensibly, "What happens if we counter the four seasons and generate chaotic qi?"

Consequences of needling counter to the seasons

Needle	In	Consequence
Networks	Spring	Blood and qi overflow outward, creating (shǎo qì) 少氣 *Scant Qi*
Muscles	Spring	Blood and qi circle and counterflow, creating (shàng qì) 上氣 *Hyperventilation*
Sinews/ Bones	Spring	Blood and qi pour inward, creating (fù zhàng) 腹脹 *Abdominal Distension*
Channels	Summer	Blood and qi are used up, creating (xiè yì) 解㑊 *Lassitude*
Muscles	Summer	Blood and qi are diminished within, creating (shàn kǒng) 善恐 *Tendency for Fearfulness*
Sinews/ Bones	Summer	Blood and qi counterflow upward, creating (shàn nù) 善怒 *Tendency for Anger*
Channels	Autumn	Blood and qi counterflow upward, creating (shàn wàng) 善忘 *Forgetfulness*
Networks	Autumn	Qi does not travel outward, creating (wò bú yù dòng) 臥不欲動 *Listlessness*, i.e. "lying down with no desire to move"
Sinews/ Bones	Autumn	Blood and qi scatter inside, creating (hán lì) 寒慄 *Cold Chills*
Channels	Winter	Blood and qi both disconnect, creating (mù bù míng) 目不明 *Poor Vision*
Networks	Winter	Internal qi leaks out, lingering to become (dà bì) 大痺 *Large Impediment*
Muscles	Winter	Yang qi is used up, creating (shàn wàng) 善忘 *Forgetfulness*

Finally, the Emperor summarizes five types of death prognoses from incorrectly needling the five Zang. We saw these motions in Chapter 23 already, as symptoms that manifest in the five zang.

Five Zang death prognoses

Needle enters	Die in	Movement
Heart	1 day	Burp 噫 (yī)
Liver	5 days	Speech 語 (yǔ)
Lung	3 days	Cough 欬 (ké)
Kidney	6 days	Sneeze 嚏 (tì) Yawn 欠 (qiàn)
Spleen	10 days	Swallow 吞 (tūn)

Chapter 65

Discussion on Root and Branch Pathophysiology

標本病傳論

(biāo běn bìng chuán lùn)

Chapter 65, Discussion on Root and Branch Pathophysiology, states the importance of knowing when to treat the root cause and when to treat the branch symptoms of a condition. It is primarily a discussion on general concepts, not specific conditions.

When to treat root versus branch

Treat the root 治本 (zhì běn)	Treat the branch 治標 (zhì biāo)
First *Disease* and then *Counterflow*	
First *Counterflow* and then *Disease*	
First *Cold* and then *Disease*	
First *Disease* and then *Cold*	
First *Heat* and then *Disease*	

	First *Heat* and then *Middle Fullness*
First *Disease* and then *Diarrhea*	
First *Diarrhea* and then *Disease*	
First *Middle Fullness* and then *Vexation*	
	Constipation or *Urine Retention*
No *Constipation* or *Urine Retention*	

General treatment principles for excess and deficiency

If the condition is caused by (yǒu yú) 有餘 "excess," treat the root first, then the branch. If the condition is caused by (bù zú) 不足 "deficiency," treat the branch first, then the root.

The second half of the chapter discusses general pathophysiology, with prognoses for death date and time.

Hallmark symptoms of each Zang

Heart	Lung	Liver	Spleen	Kidney
Heart Pain 心痛 (xīn tòng)	*Panting* 喘 (chuǎn) *Cough* 欬 (ké)	*Vertigo* 頭目眩 (tóu mù xuàn) *Rib/Armpit Fullness* 脇支滿 (xié zhī mǎn)	*Body Pain* 身痛 (shēn tòng) *Body Heaviness* 體重 (tǐ zhòng) *Abdominal Distension* 腹脹 (fù zhàng)	*Hypogastric Pain* 少腹痛 (shào fù tòng) *Low Back Pain* 腰痛 (yāo tòng) *Shin Soreness* 脛酸 (jìng suān)

Pathogenesis and prognoses of each Zang's disease

Disease	Initial symptom/s	Subsequent symptoms (number of days)	Death within	Time of death
Heart	*Heart Pain* 心痛 (xīn tòng)	*Cough* (1) 欬 (ké) *Rib/Armpit Pain* (3) 脇支痛 (xié zhī tòng) *No Throughput* (5) 閉塞不通 (bì sè bù tōng) *Body Pain/Heaviness* (5) 身痛體重 (shēn tòng tǐ zhòng)	3 days	Midnight in winter, noon in summer
Lung	*Panting* 喘 (chuǎn) *Cough* 欬 (ké)	*Rib/Armpit Fullness/Pain* (3) 脇支滿痛 (xié zhī mǎn tòng) *Body Heaviness/Pain* (1) 身重體痛 (shēn zhòng tǐ tòng) *Distension* (5) 脹 (zhàng)	10 days	Sunset in winter, sunrise in summer
Liver	*Vertigo* 頭目眩 (tóu mù xuàn) *Rib/Armpit Fullness* 脇支痛 (xié zhī mǎn)	*Distension* (3) 脹 (zhàng) *Body Heaviness/Pain* (5) 身重體痛 (shēn zhòng tǐ tòng) *Lumbar/Hypogastric Pain* 腰脊少腹痛 (yāo jǐ shào fù tòng) *Shin Soreness* (3) 脛酸 (jìng suān)	3 days	Sunset in winter, breakfast in summer
Spleen	*Body Pain* 身痛 (shēn tòng) *Body Heaviness* 體重 (tǐ zhòng)	*Distension* (1) 脹 (zhàng) *Hypogastric/Lumbar Pain* (2) 少腹腰脊痛 (shào fù yāo jǐ tòng) *Shin Soreness* (2) 脛酸 (jìng suān) *Back Sinew Pain* (3) 背脊筋痛 (bèi lǚ jīn tòng)[143] *Urinary Blockage* (3) 小便閉 (xiǎo biàn bì)	10 days	Bedtime in winter, dinnertime in summer

Kidney	*Hypogastric/Lumbar Pain* 少腹腰脊痛 (shào fù yāo jǐ tòng) *Calf Soreness* 胻痠 (héng suān)	*Back Sinew Pain* (3) 背脊筋痛 (bèi lǚ jīn tòng)[144] *Urinary Blockage* (3) 小便閉 (xiǎo biàn bì) *Abdominal Distension* (+3) 腹脹 (fù zhàng) *Rib/Armpit Pain* (+3) 脇支痛 (xié zhī tòng)	3 days	Morning in winter, afternoon in summer
Stomach	*Distension* 脹 (zhàng) *Fullness* 滿 (mǎn)	*Hypogastric/Lumbar Pain* (5) 少腹腰脊痛 (shào fù yāo jǐ tòng) *Calf Soreness* (5) 胻痠 (héng suān) *Back Sinew Pain* (3) 背脊筋痛 (bèi lǚ jīn tòng)[145] *Urinary Blockage* (3) 小便閉 (xiǎo biàn bì) *Body Heaviness* (5) 身體重 (shēn tǐ zhòng)	6 days	After midnight in winter, before sunset in summer
Bladder	*Urinary Blockage* 小便閉 (xiǎo biàn bì)	*Hypogastric Distension* (5) 少腹脹 (shào fù zhàng) *Lumbar Pain* (5) 腰脊痛 (yāo jǐ tòng) *Calf Soreness* (5) 胻痠 (héng suān) *Abdominal Distension* (1) 腹脹 (fù zhàng) *Body Pain* (+1) 體痛 (tǐ tòng)	2 days	Cocks crow in winter, late afternoon in summer

"If the pathophysiology follows the chart above, [the practitioner] may predict a death date, but may not needle. After [the disease] stops at one Zang, and spreads to three or four Zang, then it is okay to needle." According to Unschuld, this has something to do with the condition skipping a Zang in its development.

Note on Chapters 66–74: Among scholars of classical Chinese medicinal texts, many including Henry McCann, Sabine Wilms, and Paul Unschuld agree that Chapters 66–71 and 74 were added to the original text of the *Sùwèn* by Wáng Bīng 王冰, who collected and annotated the text in the Táng Dynasty 唐朝 (ca. 762).

An earlier edition was being annotated by Quán Wénqǐ 全文起 in the Nánběi Dynasty 南北朝 (ca. 420–589), but that edition has been lost.

Wáng Bīng's is considered the definitive version. He may have referenced Quán's version, or an unpublished version from his teacher, known as *Zhāng Gōng Mì Běn* 《張公秘本》 Master Zhang's Secret Folio.

Additionally, the texts of Chapter 72 and 73 were written by Liú Wēnshū 劉溫舒 of the Sòng Dynasty 宋朝 (ca. 1098). In the Wáng Bīng edition (ca. 672), only the titles of Chapters 72 and 73 were listed, as (wáng) 亡 "destroyed," or lost. Liú's version claimed they were merely (yí) 遺 "misplaced," or apocryphal. The apocryphal text ascribed to Liú Wēnshū is not included in Paul Unschuld's annotated translation.

Chapters 66–74 were not included in my original doctoral capstone. These chapters cover chronobiology and divination, also known as (wǔ yùn liù qì) 五運六氣, the "five evolutive phases and six climatic factors."

Big Discussion on Sky Origin Records

天元紀大論

(tiān yuán jì dà lùn)

Chapter 66, Big Discussion on Sky Origin Records, introduces a new character named Guǐyú Qū 鬼臾區, who introduces the Emperor to the basics of chronobiology. The Emperor begins with a question about the observable signs of three yin and three yang that is almost the same as the first line of Chapter 6, paragraph 2. Guiyu Qu answers with the first lines of Chapter 5 which define yin and yang, and adds the following information.

Definitions of 化 (huà), 變 (biàn), 神 (shén), 聖 (shèng)

Things generated/born = Transformation
物生 (wù shēng) = 化 (huà)

Things reaching their extreme polarity/end = Change
物極 (wù jí) = 變 (biàn)

Yin and Yang cannot be measured = God 陰陽不測 (yīn yáng bú cè) = 神 (shén)	
Shén-spirit Function cannot be formulated = Sage 神用無方 (shén yòng wú fāng) = 聖 (shèng)	

Much of this chapter appears to be quoted from Chapter 5, Big Discussion on Yin Yang Reflection Images. I did not translate Chapter 5 line by line, but looking at Chapter 66, I see some of the information I skipped over can be organized as follows.

Functions of change and transformation in sky, human, and land from Chapter 66

Function of change and transformation	in Sky	in Human	Land
is ~	(xuán) 玄 Darkness	(dào) 道 Way	(huà) 化 Transformation
which generates	(shén) 神 Spirit	(zhì) 智 Wit	(wǔ wèi) 五味 Five Flavors

Shén-spirit in sky and on land

In sky is ~ 在天為 (zài tiān wéi)	Wind 風 (fēng)	Heat 熱 (rè)	Damp 濕 (shī)	Dry 燥 (zào)	Cold 寒 (hán)	Qi 氣 (qì)
On land is ~ 在地為 (zài dì wéi)	Wood 木 (mù)	Fire 火 (huǒ)	Earth 土 (tǔ)	Metal 金 (jīn)	Water 水 (shuǐ)	Form 形 (xíng)

The mutual interaction of form and qi creates everything. However, sky and land (i.e. weather and geography) are the up and down of everything. Left and right are the paths of yin and yang. Water and fire are the signals of yin and yang. Metal and wood are the end and beginning of generation. The amount of qi matches the abundance and decline of the form (i.e. the body) above and below.

The Emperor says, "[I would like to hear of] how the five evolutive phases govern seasons."

Guiyu Qu answers with a quote from the *Tàishǐ Tiānyuán Cè* 《太史天元冊》 <u>Book of Most Historical Sky Origins</u> about nine stars and seven planets.

The Emperor then asks about the abundance and scarcity of qi and form, and Guiyu Qu says, "The qi of yin and yang have more or less, that is why we say three yin and three yang. The form has abundance and scarcity, that is why we say the treatment of five elements each have too much and not enough." He then explains how prognosis relates to excess and deficiency.

The Emperor asks about mutual summons from above and below.

Guiyu Qu states, "Cold, Summerheat, Dry, Damp, Wind, and Fire are the sky's yin and yang. The three yin and three yang reflect it above. Wood, fire, earth, metal, water, and fire* are the land's yin and yang. Generation, growth, transformation, withdrawal and storage reflect it below. Sky generates with yang and grows with yin. Land kills with yang and hides with yin. The sky has yin and yang, and so does the land." He explains the yin within yang and yang within yin with a description of how the yin and yang of sky and land reflect the qi of land every five (suì) 歲, and the qi of sky every six (jì) 暮.

The Emperor asks whether (zhōu) 周 "circuits" and (jì) 紀 "records" can be predetermined. Guiyu Qu answers, "The sky has six as its (jié) 節 "nodes". The land has five as its (zhì) 制 "limits". One zhōu-circuit of sky's qì-node is six (jì) 暮, known as one (bèi) 備. One zhōu-circuit of land's jì-record is five (suì) 歲." It appears that both jì and suì equal one year. Therefore, sky qi circuits every six years, and land qi circuits every five years.

---

*   Fire appears twice.

Qi Bo says,* "720 qì-nodes (i.e. 30 years) make one jì-record. 1440 qì-nodes (i.e. 60 years) make one zhōu-circuit." The Emperor and Guiyu Qu discuss how this knowledge can be applied to governance of the people and treatment of the body. They go back and forth a few times with what sounds like formalized pleasantries, until the Emperor requests the essentials of chronobiology according to the (tiān gān) 天干 "10 heavenly stems" and (dì zhī) 地支 "12 earthly branches", which Guiyu Qu supplies.

Essentials of chronobiology

Year of	甲己 (jiǎ jǐ)	乙庚 (yǐ gēng)	丙辛 (bǐng xīn)	丁壬 (dīng rèn)	戊癸 (wù guǐ)	
Ruled by evolutive phase of	Earth	Metal	Water	Wood	Fire	
Year of	子午 (zǐ wǔ)	丑未 (chǒu wèi)	寅申 (yín shēn)	卯酉 (mǎo yǒu)	辰戌 (chén xū)	巳亥 (sì hài)
Converges with	Shaoyin	Taiyin	Shaoyang	Yangming	Taiyang	Jueyin

Shaoyin is known as the branch. Jueyin is known as the end.

(běn) 本 Root, also known as the (liù yuán) 六元 Six Origins

Above	Jueyin	Shaoyin	Taiyin	Shaoyang	Yangming	Taiyang
~governs	Wind qi	Heat qi	Damp qi	Ministerial Fire	Dry qi	Cold qi

The Emperor is delighted by the six yuán-origins and declares that he will have it inscribed on a jade tablet for his Golden Cabinet under the title *Tiānyuán Jì* 天元紀 <u>Sky Origin Record</u>.

---

* This statement is preceded by a comment about imperial versus ministerial fire which I have omitted.

Big Discussion on the Five Evolutive Phase Movements

五運行大論

(wǔ yùn xíng dà lùn)

Chapter 67, Big Discussion on the Five Evolutive Phase Movements, is a conversation between the Yellow Emperor, Guiyu Qu, and Qi Bo. The Emperor calls Qi Bo (tiān shī) 天師 "Sky Master," a Daoist title we saw him use in Chapter 1. He calls Guiyu Qu (fū zǐ) 夫子,* an honorific for an educated man. They begin by revisiting the conversation from the end of Chapter 66, filling Qi Bo in on which of the five elements and six channels govern which years. Guiyu Qu asks Qi Bo why the

---

* 夫子 (fū zǐ): this is the "fucius" part of Confucius, whose real name was Kǒng Qiū 孔丘. Confucius is a transliteration of (kǒng fū zǐ) 孔夫子 "Master Kong." Apparently, any well-educated man may be referred to as (fū zǐ) 夫子, but in colloquial Chinese today when people say (fū zǐ) 夫子 they usually mean Confucius.

divination of chronobiology sometimes fails to match yin and yang. Qi Bo quotes himself from the beginning of Chapter 6.

Energetics of the constellations

The Emperor says, "I would like to hear of the beginning."

Qi Bo says, "Excellent question!" I browsed the text of *Tàishǐ Tiānyuán Cè* 《太始天元冊》 <u>Book of Most Historical Sky Origins</u>, which states the following:

~ qi of sky	Passes through constellations[146]	Heavenly Stem: Constellations
Cinnabar 丹 (dān)	Cowherd 牛 (niú) Weavergirl 女 (nǚ)	戊 (wù): 軫 (zhěn) Chariot 角 (jiǎo) Dragonhorn 壁 (bì) Eastwall 奎 (kuí) Tigerlegs
Golden-yellow 黅 (jīn)	Dragonheart 心 (xīn) Dragontail 尾 (wěi)	己 (jǐ): 軫 (zhěn) Chariot 角 (jiǎo) Dragonhorn 壁 (bì) Eastwall 奎 (kuí) Tigerlegs
Blue-gray 蒼 (cāng)	Rooftop 危 (wéi) Room 室 (shì) Willowbeak 柳 (liǔ) Ghosts 鬼 (guǐ)	
Plain 素 (sù)	Dragonthroat 亢 (kàng) Dragonfoot 氐 (dī) Tigerfuzz 昴 (mǎo) Fork 畢 (bì)	
Darkness 玄 (xuán)	Open-net 張 (zhāng) Wings 翼 (yì) Garment-train 婁 (lóu) Stomach 胃 (wèi)	

"These are the doors and windows of heaven and earth, the beginning of (hòu) 候 "waits" and the birth of (dào) 道 "the Way". They must not be made impassable."

Energetics of directions

The Emperor asks next about up and down versus right and left.

Qi Bo says that a year's up and down reveal where yin and yang are. As for left and right:

~ above	Left	Right	~ below
Jueyin	Shaoyin	Taiyang	Shaoyang
Shaoyin	Taiyin	Jueyin	Yangming
Taiyin	Shaoyang	Shaoyin	Taiyang
Shaoyang	Yangming	Taiyin	Jueyin
Yangming	Taiyang	Shaoyang	Shaoyin
Taiyang	Jueyin	Yangming	Taiyin

Above is what's known as facing north and determining (wèi) 位 "positions". Below is what's known as facing south and determining (wèi) 位 "positions".

Positions and Directions and disease

Upper and lower communicate with each other. Cold and heat approach each other. If qi aligns, then harmony. If they do not align, then disease [happens].

I think upper here means the sky/climatic factors and lower means the land/evolutive phases, but I am not sure.

The Emperor says, "Why does disease [sometimes] occur [when] qi is aligned?"

Qi Bo says, "That is when the lower approaches the upper, not in the appropriate position."

The Emperor says, "What of movement and stillness?"

Qi Bo says, "Upper travels to the right. Lower travels to the left. Left and right circuit the sky and then meet again."

The Emperor says, "I heard Guiyu Qu say, 'That which reflects the land is still.' However, you say the lower travels to the left. I do not understand what you are talking about. I would like to hear of how/what is generated."

Qi Bo says, "The movement and stillness of sky and land, the departure and return of five elements, though observed by Guiyu Qu [as an astrologer], cannot be entirely illuminated. The functions of change and transformation, sky dangles (xiàng) 象 'phenomena,' land completes (xíng) 形 'form,' the seven stars and planets* weft the void, the five elements beautify the land. Land carries the birth and completion of form and categories. Void† arrays the essence and qi that reflect heaven. The movements of form and essence are connected like roots and leaves on branches. Though distant, looking up and observing the phenomena yields knowledge."

The Emperor then asks whether land is lower. Qi Bo says, "Land is below humans, the center of the (tài xū) 太虛 'great void'."

How the six big qi affect the land

Big qi 大氣 (dà qì)	Action	Location	Effect on land
Dryness 燥 (zào)	Dries 乾 (gān)	Above 上 (shàng)	Dry 乾 (gān)
Summerheat 暑 (shǔ)	Steams 蒸 (zhēng)	Above 上 (shàng)	Hot 熱 (rè)
Wind 風 (fēng)	Moves 動 (dòng)	Below 下 (xià)	Moves 動 (dòng)

---

* 七曜 (qī yào): seven shining celestial bodies, i.e. the sun, the moon, Venus, Jupiter, Mercury, Mars, and Saturn.

† 虛 (xū): void, same character as empty, vacuous, or deficient.

Dampness 濕 (shī)	Moistens 潤 (rùn)	Center 中 (zhōng)	Muddy 泥 (ní)
Cold 寒 (hán)	Hardens 堅 (jiān)	Below 下 (xià)	Cracks 裂 (liè)
Fire 火 (huǒ)	Warms 溫 (wēn)	Wanders between 游間 (yóu jiān)	Harden 固 (gù)

Pulse, between qi, and more five element diagnosis

The Emperor then asks how one might observe the qi of sky and land. Qi Bo quotes a book on pulse techniques called *Mài Fǎ* 《脈法》 <u>Pulse Method</u>, which states that "the changes of sky and land may not be diagnosed through the pulse."

The Emperor then asks about something called (jiān qì) 閒 氣 "between qi," which is apparently the belief that the qi of the year affects prognoses. Between qi is covered in detail in Chapter 74.

The rest of the chapter is devoted to the five elements, mostly a reiteration of information from Chapter 5, which is covered in the table on the generating cycle on page 44. I have collected the new concepts unique to Chapter 67 in the following table.

	Wood	Fire	Earth	Metal	Water
Nature 性 (xìng)	Ruckus 喧 (xuān)	Summerheat 暑 (shǔ)	Quietude 靜 (jìng)	Coolness 涼 (liáng)	Shudder 凜 (lǐn)
Virtue 德 (dé)	Harmony 和 (hé)	Revelation 顯 (xiǎn)	Immersion 濡 (rú)	Clarity 清 (qīng)	Cold 寒 (hán)
Function	Movement	Restlessness	Transformation	Harden	LOST
Transformation	Glory	Luxuriance	Increscence	Restraint	Silence
Creature	Furry	Feathery	Naked	Shelled	Scaly
Governance	Scatter	Brightness	Quietude	Force	Quietude
Command	Announce Release	Depress Steam	Wind Rain	Fog Dew	LOST LOST
Change	Break Pull	Inflame Glitter	Move Pour	Silence Kill	Freeze Chill
Calamity[147]	Fall[148]	Roast/Scald	Saturate/Flood	Age/Drop	Ice/Hail

Big Discussion on the Six Subtle Purposes

六微旨大論

(liù wēi zhǐ dà lùn)

Chapter 68, Big Discussion on the Six Subtle Purposes, appears to be about measurements of time. The first passage is the Emperor exclaiming about the astonishing distance of the Way of Heaven, "As if welcoming floating clouds, like viewing a deep abyss. Abysses, however deep, may yet be measured, but who knows where the clouds end?*" He refers to Qi Bo's repeated admonishments to respect (tiān dào) 天道 "Heaven's Way," and asks for explications of the (tiān zhī dào) 天之道 "Way of Heaven/Sky." I think (tiān) 天 here means the passage of time, and what happens in the world accordingly.

---

*   「嗚呼遠哉, 天之道也, 如迎浮雲, 若視深淵, 視深淵尚可測, 迎浮雲莫知其
      極。」(wū hū yuǎn zāi, tiān zhī dào yě, rú yíng fú yún, ruò shì shēn yuān,
      shì shēn yuān shàng kě cè, yíng fú yún mò zhī qí jí).

Qi Bo compliments the Emperor's questions and answers that the chronology of sky determines the seasons of abundance and decline.

The seasonal nodes

Qi Bo says, Above and below are (wèi) 位 "positions." Left and right are (jì) 紀 "records."

Right of	Governed by
Shaoyang	Yangming
Yangming	Taiyang
Taiyang	Jueyin
Jueyin	Shaoyin
Shaoyin	Taiyin
Taiyin	Shaoyang

This is known as the branch* of qi.† Therefore it is said, "Due to the chronology of sky (i.e. time?), the seasons of abundance and decline, the movement and positions of light, stand straight‡ and wait."§

---

* 標 (biāo): The distal ends of wood (SWJZ), most often translated as "branch."

† I have omitted a line here about awaiting the south-facing cover/entirety:「蓋南面而待也。」(gài nán miàn ér dài yě)

‡ 正立 (zhèng lì): [to] stand upright.

§ 「此所謂氣之標, 蓋南面而待也。故曰: 因天之序, 盛衰之時, 移光定位, 正立而待之, 此之謂也。」(cǐ suǒ wèi qì zhī biāo, gài nán miàn ér dài yě. gù yuē: yīn tiān zhī xū, shèng shuāi zhī shí, yí guāng dìng wèi, zhèng lì ér dài zhī, cǐ zhī wèi yě).

Root, middle, and climatic factors

Above	Governed by ~ qi	Middle (jiàn)見 "Sight"
Shaoyang	Fire	Jueyin
Yangming	Dry	Taiyin
Taiyang	Cold	Shaoyin
Jueyin	Wind	Shaoyang
Shaoyin	Heat	Taiyang
Taiyin	Damp	Yangming

This is the root. Below the root is the Sight* of middle; below the Sight is the branch of qi. When the root and branch are not the same, differences reflect in the qi.

Chronobiological definitions

Harmony 和 (hé)	[Qi] arrives at its time
Deficiency 不及 (bù jí)	Coming qi does not arrive at its time
Excess 有餘 (yǒu yú)	Coming qi arrives before its time
Submissive 順 (shùn)	Echoes/Reflects/Answers 應 (yìng)
Rebellious 逆 (nì)	Refutes/Rejects 否 (fǒu) Creates change, which leads to disease

Life echoes things. Pulse echoes qi.

---

* 見 (jiàn): Sight (SWJZ), literally a pictograph of an eyeball turned sideways with legs.

Geography echoes the positions of the six qì-nodes with the generating/insulting cycle

This section reads like a dance manual, or a board game rulebook: "To the right of (xiǎn míng) 顯明 'Revealing Brightness' is the position of imperial fire. To the right of imperial fire, back up one step, ministerial fire governs it. Take one more step, earth qi governs it. Take one more step, metal qi governs it. Take one more step, water qi governs it. Take one more step, wood qi governs it. Take one more step, imperial fire governs it. Below ministerial fire, water qi holds it up. Positioned below water, earth qi holds it up. Positioned below earth, wind qi holds it up. Positioned below wind, metal qi holds it up. Positioned below metal, fire qi holds it up. Below imperial fire, yin essence holds it up." When we look more carefully at this, it describes the generating cycle and the reverse of the controlling cycle.

The Emperor next asks about abundance and decline, class (noble versus base), pathogen/s striking, positions shifting,* and steps.

---

* 位之易 (wèi zhī yì): "Change/shift of position." This is the character (yì) 易 "change" as in the I Ching, or Book of Changes..

Beginning and end, earliness and lateness of the six climatic factors by year*

Year of	60-day[149] qi-cycle of						Sky's number 天之數 (tiān zhī shù)
	Beginning 初 (chū)	Two 二 (èr)	Three 三 (sān)	Four 四 (sì)	Five 五 (wǔ)	Six 六 (liù)	
甲子 (jiǎ zǐ)	water clock 1-87.5	87.6-75	76-62.5	62.6-50	51-37.5	37.6-25	Beginning Six 初六
乙丑 (yǐ chǒu)	26-12.5	12.6-water clock 100	1-87.5	87.6-75	76-62.5	62.6-40	Six Two 六二
丙寅 (bǐng yín)	51-37.5	37.6-25	26-12.5	12.6-water clock 100	1-87.5	87.6-75	Six Three 六三
丁卯 (dīng mǎo)	76-62.5	62.6-50	51-37.5	37.6-25	26-12.5	12.6-water clock 100	Six Four 六四
戊辰 (wù chén)	1-and so on...						

(suì hòu) 歲候 Year waits

Week	1	2	3	4	5
Sky's qi begins at ~ (kè) 刻	1	26	51	76	Start over at 1

This is known as 1 (jì) 紀 "record."

Similar years

寅 (yín)	卯 (mǎo)	辰 (chén)	巳 (sì)
午 (wǔ)	未 (wèi)	申 (shēn)	酉 (yǒu)
戌 (xū)	亥 (hài)	子 (zǐ)	丑 (chǒu)

Functional applications and qi exchange

The Emperor asks about (yòng) 用 ...uses? functions? Maybe functional applications.

Qi Bo answers, "Speaking of sky, go for the root. Speaking of land, go for the position. Speaking of human, go for qi exchange."

The Emperor asks, "What is qi exchange?"

Qi Bo answers, "Above and below are positions. Qi exchange is the middle, where humans dwell. Therefore it is said, 'Above the (tiān shū) 天樞 "sky pivot"* is governed by sky qi. Below the (tiān shū) 天樞 "sky pivot" is governed by land qi. At the separation of qi exchange is human qi, which everything[†] obeys.'"[‡]

---

* 天樞 (tiān shū): Sky Pivot is the name of the star that connects the handle and scoop of the Big Dipper constellation. **Acu Trivia**! Also the name of acupoint St25.

† 萬物 (wàn wù): ten thousand things, i.e. everything.

‡ 由 (yóu): originally a pictograph depicting a seed sprouting from a field, (yóu) 由 can mean to sprout, to obey/follow, or to pass through.

Ascending/Descending sky and land qi

The next passage goes into the ascending and descending qualities of sky qi and land qi, and the uses thereof. I lose the thread of it, but at one point Qi Bo returns to the concept that things are born from the action of (huà) 化 "transformation" and things end due to the action of (biàn) 變 "change." Without (shēng) 升 "ascent" and (jiàng) 降 "descent," (shēng) 生 "generation" and (huà) 化 "transformation" cannot occur. This chapter ends with the Emperor asking, "Is there [such a thing as] no generation and no transformation?"

Qi Bo says, "Great question. Only true humans* converge into sameness with the Way."

The Emperor says, "Ah."

---

* 真人 (zhēn rén).

Big Discussion on Qi Exchange Changes

氣交變大論

(qì jiāo biàn dà lùn)

Chapter 69, Big Discussion on Qi Exchange Changes, offers details on the five evolutive phases in years of excess, years of insufficiency, changes reflected in the four seasons and the five planets, and the movements of virtue, transformation, governance, and command.

The chapter begins with a number of formal pleasantries which leads to Qi Bo quoting the *Shàng Jīng* 《上經》 Upper Classic:

夫道者,
(fū dào zhě,)
Of the Way,

上知天文,
(shàng zhī tiān wén,)
knowing astronomy above,

下知地理,
(xià zhī dì lǐ,)
knowing geography below,

中知人事,
(zhōng zhī rén shì,)
[and] knowing human affairs in the middle,

可以長久。
(kě yǐ cháng jiǔ.)
make sustainability possible.

Excess of five evolutive phases*

Year of excess	Wood
~ qi flows and moves	Wind
~ receives pathogens	Spleen Earth
People [get these] diseases 民病 (mín bìng)	*Lienteric Diarrhea* 飧泄 (sūn xiè) *Reduced Appetite* 食減 (shí jiǎn) *Body Heaviness* 體重 (tǐ zhòng) *Vexation Grievance* 煩冤 (fán yuān) *Borborygmus* 腸鳴 (cháng míng) *Abdominal/Propping Fullness* 腹支滿 (fù zhī mǎn)

---

* Qi Bo's answer to the Emperor's question about the excess of five evolutive phases actually includes a lot of weather forecasts for each year as well, most of which I have skipped over or relegated to footnotes. Not purely because I do not understand them; I believe that climate change has made the predictions of ancient civilizations (e.g. the Chinese five-phase six-conformations, the Mayan calendar predictions) unreliable.

Reflects [planet]	Jupiter
Extreme cases: signs and symptoms	*Frustration with Tendency to Anger* 忽忽善怒 (hū hū shàn nù) *Dizziness Veiling* 眩冒 (xuàn mào) *Vertex Disease* 巔疾 (diān jí)
	Rib Pain with Extreme Vomiting 脇痛而吐甚 (xié tòng ér tù shèn)[150]
If ~ ends, death	"Rushing Yang" (chōng yáng) 衝陽 St42 Dorsal Pulse
Reflects [planet]	Venus

Year of excess	**Fire**
~ qi flows and moves	Inflamed summerheat 炎暑 (yán shǔ)
~ receives pathogens	Metal Lung
People [get these] diseases	*Ague* 瘧 (nuè) *Scant Qi* 少氣 (shǎo qì) *Cough, Panting* 欬喘 (ké chuǎn) *Blood Upwelling,*[151] i.e. epistaxis, hematemesis, hemoptysis 血溢 (xiě yì) *Bloody Diarrhea*, i.e. hematochezia 血泄 (xiě xiè) *Copious Watery Diarrhea* 注下 (zhù xià) *Esophageal Dryness* 嗌燥 (yì gān) *Deafness* 耳聾 (ěr lóng) *Center Heat* 中熱 (zhōng rè) *Shoulder/Upper Back Heat* 肩背熱 (jiān bèi rè)

Year of excess	Fire
Reflects	Mars
Extreme cases: signs and symptoms	*Chest/Center Pain* 胸中痛 (xiōng zhōng tòng) *Rib/Propping Fullness* 脇支滿 (xié zhī mǎn) *Rib Pain* 脇痛 (xié tòng) *Lateral Chest/Upper Back/Scapular Pain* 膺背肩胛間痛 (yīng bèi jiān jiǎ jiān tòng) *Bilateral Medial Arm Pain* 兩臂內痛 (liǎng bì nèi tòng) *Body Hot* 身熱 (shēn rè) with *Bone Pain* 骨痛 (gǔ tòng) *Immersion*, i.e. infection 浸淫 (jìn yín)
Reflects	Mercury
Triumph of Shaoyin Shaoyang	*Forgetfulness with Delirium/Mania* 譫妄狂越 (zhān wàng kuáng yuè) Panting Cough with Audible breathing 欬喘息鳴 (ké chuǎn xī míng) *Blood Upwelling/Nonstop Diarrhea* 血溢泄不已 (xiě yì xiè bù yǐ)
If ~ ends, death	"Great Abyss" (tài yuān) 太淵 Lu9 Radial Pulse
Reflects	Mars

Year of excess	Earth
~ qi flows and moves	Rain damp
~ receives pathogens	Kidney Water
People [get these] diseases	*Abdominal Pain* 腹痛 (fù tòng) *Cool Reversal*, i.e. cold feet 清厥 (qīng jué) *Lack of Joy* 意不樂 (yì bú lè) *Body Heaviness* 體重 (tǐ zhòng) *Vexation Grievance* 煩冤 (fán yuān)
Reflects	Saturn
Extreme cases: signs and symptoms	*Muscle Atrophy* 肌肉萎 (jī ròu wěi) *Leg Atrophy* 足痿 (zú wěi) with *Inability to Contract* 不收 (bù shōu) *Tendency to Cramp [when] Walking* 行善瘛 (xíng shàn chì) *Foot/Sole Pain* 腳下痛 (jiǎo xià tòng) *Rheum* expressed as 飲發 (yǐn fā) • *Middle Fullness* 中滿 (zhōng mǎn) • *Reduced Appetite* 食減 (shí jiǎn) • *Inability to Lift Limbs* 四支不舉 (sì zhī bù jǔ) *Abdominal Fullness* 腹滿 (fù mǎn) *Loose Stools/Diarrhea* 溏泄 *(táng xiè)Borborygmus* 腸鳴 (cháng míng) with *Extreme Precipitation* 反下甚 (fǎn xià shèn)[152]
If ~ ends, death	"Great Stream" (tài xī) 太溪 K3 Posterior Tibial Pulse
Reflects	Jupiter
Year of excess	**Metal**
~ qi flows and moves	Dry qi

~ receives pathogens	Liver Wood
People [get these] diseases	*Bilateral Rib/Hypochondriac/Hypogastric Pain* 兩脇下少腹痛 (liǎng xié xià shào fù tòng) *Eyes Red and Painful* 目赤痛 (mù chì tòng) *Sores at Canthus* 眥瘍 (zì yáng) *Inability to Hear* 耳無所聞 (ěr wú suǒ wén)
	Body Heaviness 體重 (tǐ zhòng) *Vexation Grievance* 煩冤 (fán yuān) *Chest Pain* 胸痛 (xiōng tòng) *Radiating to Upper Back* 引背 (yǐn bèi) *Bilateral Rib Fullness with Pain Radiating to Hypogastrium* 兩脇滿且痛引少腹 (liǎng xié mǎn qiě tòng yǐn shào fù)[153]
Reflects	Venus
Extreme cases: signs and symptoms	*Panting Cough* 喘欬 (chuǎn ké) *Counterflow Qi* 逆氣 (nì qì) *Shoulder/Upper Back Pain* 肩背痛 (jiān bèi tòng) *Sacrum, Genital, Buttock, Knee, Hip, Calf, Shin and Leg Disease* 尻陰股膝髀腨胻足皆病 (kāo yīn gǔ xī bì shuǎn héng zú jiē bìng)
	Violent Pain 暴痛 (bào tòng) *Torso/Ribs Unable to Extend/Laterally Rotate* 胠脇不可反側 (qū xié bù kě fǎn cè) *[If] Cough/Counterflow extreme, then Blood Upwelling* 欬逆甚而血溢 (ké nì shèn ér xiě yì) [154]
If ~ ends, death	"Great Rushing" (tài chōng) 太衝 Lv3 Pulse
Reflects	Mars
Year of excess	**Water**
~ qi flows and moves	Cold qi

~ receives pathogens	Heart Fire
People [get these] diseases	*Body Hot* 身熱 (shēn rè) *Vexation* 煩 (fán) *Heart Restless/Palpitations* 心躁悸 (xīn zào jì) *Yin Reversal* 陰厥 (yīn jué) *Upper, Lower, Middle Cold* 上下中寒 (shàng xià zhōng hán) *Delirium* 譫妄 (zhān wàng) *Heart Pain*, i.e. angina 心痛 (xīn tòng)
Reflects	Mercury
Extreme cases: signs and symptoms	*Abdomen Enlarged* 腹大 (fù dà) *Shin Swelling* 脛腫 (jìng zhǒng) *Panting Cough* 喘欬 (chuǎn ké) *Night Sweats* 寢汗 (qǐn hàn) with *Abhorrence of Wind* 憎風 (zēng fēng)
Reflects	Saturn
Triumph of Taiyang	*Abdominal Fullness* 腹滿 (fù mǎn) *Borborygmus* 腸鳴 (cháng míng) *Loose Stools/Diarrhea* 溏泄 (táng xiè) *Indigestion* 食不化 (shí bú huà) *Thirst* 渴 (kě) with *Frenetic Veiling* 妄冒 (wàng mào)
If ~ ends, death	"Spirit Door" (shén mén) 神門 H7 Ulnar Pulse
Reflects	Mars and Mercury

The Emperor then asks about the insufficiency of five evolutive phases.

Year of insufficiency	Wood
People [get these] diseases	*Gallbladder/Subaxillary/Rib Pain* 中清胠脇痛 (zhōng qīng qū xié tòng) *Hypogastric Pain* 少腹痛 (shào fù tòng) *Borborygmus* 腸鳴 (cháng míng) *Loose Stools/Diarrhea* 溏泄 (táng xiè)
Reflects	Venus
Triumph of Yangming	No symptoms listed
Reflects	Venus and Saturn
Retaliation	*Cold Heat* 寒熱 (hán rè) *Sores* 瘡 (chuāng) *Ulcers* 瘍 (yáng) *Rash* 痱 (fèi) *Pustules* 胗 (zhēn) *Carbuncles* 癰 (yōng) *Acne* 痤 (cuó)
Reflects	Mars and Venus
~ receives pathogens	Spleen Earth
Symptoms	*Cough* 欬 (ké) with *Nasal Congestion* 衄 (nù)
Reflects	Mercury and Venus
Year of insufficiency	**Fire**

People [get these] diseases	*Chest/Center Pain* 胸中痛 (xiōng zhōng tòng) *Ribs/Propping Fullness* 脇支滿 (xié zhī mǎn) *Bilateral Rib Pain* 兩脇痛 (liǎng xié tòng) *Lateral Chest/Upper Back/Scapular Pain and Medial Arm Pain* 膺背肩胛間痛及兩臂內痛 (yīng bèi jiān jiǎ jiān tòng jí liǎng bèi nèi tòng) *Depression Veiling* 鬱冒 (yù mào) *Blurry Vision* 朦昧 (méng mèi) *Heart Pain* 心痛 (xīn tòng) *Violent Aphonia* 暴瘖 (bào yīn) *Chest/Abdomen Enlarged* 胸腹大 (xiōng fù dà) *Hypochondria Radiating to Lower/Upper Back Pain* 脇下與腰背相引而痛 (xié xià yǔ yāo bèi xiāng yǐn ér tòng) *Flexion without Extension* 屈不能伸 (qū bù néng shēn)[155] *Hip and Thigh as if Separated* 髖髀如別 (kuān bì rú bié)
Reflects	Mars and Mercury
Retaliation	*Duck Slop*, i.e. loose stools? 鶩溏 (wù táng) *Abdominal Fullness* 腹滿 (fù mǎn) *Inability to Eat or Drink* 食飲不下 (shí yǐn bú xià) *Cold Strike Borborygmus* 寒中腸鳴 (hán zhòng cháng míng) *Outpour Diarrhea* 泄注 (xiè zhù) *Abdominal Pain* 腹痛 (fù tòng) *Violent Contraction, Atrophy, Impediment* 暴攣痿痺 (bào luán wěi bì) *Loss of Leg Function* 足不任身 (zú bú rèn shēn)
Reflects	Saturn and Mercury

Year of insufficiency	Earth
People [get these] diseases	*Lienteric Diarrhea* 殖泄 (sūn xiè) *Sudden Chaos* 霍亂 (huò luàn) *Body Heaviness* 體重 (tǐ zhòng) *Abdominal Pain* 腹痛 (fù tòng) *Sinews/Bones Forced Labor??* 筋骨繇復 (jīn gǔ yáo fù) *Muscle Twitch/Soreness* 肌肉瞤酸 (jī ròu rún suān) *Tendency to Anger* 善怒 (shàn nù)
Reflects	Jupiter and Saturn
Retaliation	*Chest/Ribs Violent Pain* 胸脇暴痛 (xiōng xié bào tòng) *Radiating downward to Hypogastrium* 下引少腹 (xià yǐn shào fù) *Tendency to Sigh* 善太息 (shàn tài xī) *Reduced Appetite* 食少 (shí shǎo) *Loss of Taste* 失味 (shī wèi)
Reflects	Venus and Jupiter
Triumph of Jueyin	No symptoms listed
Reflects	Jupiter[156]

Year of insufficiency	Metal
People [get these] diseases	*[at] Shoulders/Upper Back* 肩背 (jiān bèi) *Diplopia* 瞀重 (mào chóng) *Nasal Congestion* 鼽 (qiú) *Sneezing* 嚏 (tì) *Hematochezia* 血便 (xiě biàn) *Copious Watery Diarrhea* 注下 (zhù xià) [157]

Year of insufficiency	Metal
Reflects	Venus
Retaliation	*Yin Reversal* 陰厥 (yīn jué) with *Blocked Yang* 格陽 (gé yáng) traveling upward to create *Head/Du17 Pain* 頭腦戶痛 (tóu nǎo hù tòng) and *Fontanel Expresses Heat* 顖頂發熱 (xìn dǐng fā rè)
Reflects	Mercury
Signs when cinnabar harvest fails	*Mouth Ulcers* 口瘡 (kǒu chuāng) in extreme cases *Heart Pain* 心痛 (xīn tòng)

Year of insufficiency	Water
People [get these] diseases	*Abdominal Fullness* 腹滿 (fù mǎn) *Body Heaviness* 身重 (shēn zhòng) *Soggy Diarrhea* 濡泄 (rú xiè) *Cold Sores* 寒瘍 (hán yáng) with *Watery Exudation* 流水 (liú shuǐ) *Low Back/Buttock Pain Flares* 腰股痛發 (yāo gǔ tòng fā) *Popliteal/Gastrocnemius/Buttock/Knee Dysfunction* 膕腨股膝不便 (guó ruì gǔ xī bú biàn) *Vexation Grievance* 煩冤 (fán yuān) *Leg Atrophy/Cool/Reversal* 足痿清厥 (zú wěi qīng jué) *Foot/Sole Pain* 腳下痛 (jiǎo xià tòng) in extreme cases *Dorsal [Foot] Swelling* 跗腫 (fū zhǒng)
Reflects [planet]	Mercury

Year of insufficiency	Water
Triumph of Taiyin	*Cold Ailment Below* 寒疾於下 (hán jí yú xià) in extreme cases *Abdominal Fullness* 腹滿 (fù mǎn) and *Superficial Swelling* 浮腫 (fú zhǒng)
Reflects	Saturn
Retaliation	*Periodic Complexion Changes* 面色時變 (miàn sè shí biàn) *Sinews/Bones Simultaneously Split?* 筋骨併辟 (jīn gǔ bìng pì) *Muscle Twitches/Convulsions* 肉瞤瘛 (ròu rún chì) *Blurry Vision* 目視䀮䀮 (mù shì máng máng) *Things Carelessly Crack* 物疎璺 (wù shū wèn) *Muscle Pustule Eruptions* 肌肉胗發 (jī ròu zhēn fā) *Qi Merge in Diaphragm/Middle* 氣并膈中 (qì bìng gé zhōng) *Pain at Heart/Abdomen* 痛於心腹 (tòng yú xīn fù)
Reflect	Jupiter

How the five evolutive phases are reflected in the four seasons

Insufficient year	Wood	Fire	Earth	Metal	Water
Calamity	East	South	4 (wéi) 維[158]	West	North
Zang	Liver	Heart	Spleen	Lung	Kidney
Disease locations: internal	Trunk Ribs	Chest Ribs	Heart Abdomen	Chest Ribs Shoulders Upper back	Low back Spine Bones Marrow
Disease locations: external	Gates Nodes	Channels Collaterals	Muscles Limbs	Skin Body Hair	Streams Valleys Heels Knees

The governance of the five evolutive phases act as a balance to: suppress the high, raise the low, reflect the transformed, and repeat the changed.

Then they go into the divination of sudden catastrophes, which involves virtues, transformations, governances, and commands. Most of these terms are unfamiliar territory, so I assume they have to do specifically with the chronobiology of these chapters. However, many recur in the next chapter, so I have given just the Chinese terms in this table.

Five elements: virtue, transformation, governance, command, change, and catastrophe

	East	South	Center	West	North
Generates	Wind	Heat	Damp	Dry	Cold
Generates	Wood	Fire	Earth	Metal	Water
Virtue	敷和 (fū hé)	彰顯 (zhāng xiǎn)	溽蒸 (rù zhēng)	清潔 (qīng jié)	淒滄 (qī cāng)
Transformation	生榮 (shēng róng)	蕃茂 (fán mào)	豐備 (kǎi bèi)	緊斂 (jǐn liǎn)	清謐 (qīng mì)
Governance	舒啟 (shū qǐ)	明曜 (míng yào)	安靜 (ān jìng)	勁切 (jìn qiē)	凝肅 (níng sù)
Command	Wind	Heat	Damp	Dry	Cold
Change	振發 (zhèn fā)	銷爍 (xiāo shuò)	驟注 (zhòu zhù)	肅殺 (sù shā)	凓冽 (lì liè)
Catastrophe	散落 (sàn luò)	燔焫 (fán ruò)	霖潰 (lín kuì)	蒼隕 (cāng yǔn)	Ice, snow, frost, and hail

For the rest of the chapter, the Emperor and Qi Bo discuss the discrepancies that (qì jiāo) 氣交 "Qi Exchange" may create in the virtues and transformations, governance and commands, catastrophes and calamities, and changes. At the end of the chapter, the Emperor decides to put the information Qi Bo just imparted into his library (líng shì) 靈室 the "Soul Chamber," and title it *Qì Jiāo Biàn* 《氣交變》 <u>Qi Exchange Changes</u>. He plans to reread it daily out loud and promises Qi Bo not to disseminate the knowledge lightly.

Big Discussion on the Five Common Governances

五常政大論

(wǔ cháng zhèng dà lùn)

Chapter 70, Big Discussion on the Five Common Governances, details the even qi, insufficient and excess jì-records of the five phases, their effect on climate outside and within the human body, their effect on the fertility of all creatures, and the general guidelines on prescribing herbs (which we still use today).

Chinese names of years with even, insufficient, and excess five elements

Names	Wood	Fire	Earth	Metal	Water
Even[159]	敷合 (fū hé)	升明 (shēng míng)	備化 (bèi huà)	審平 (shěn píng)	靜順 (jìng shùn)
Insufficient[160]	委和 (wěi hé)	伏明 (fú míng)	卑監 (bēi jiān)	從革 (cóng gé)	涸流 (hé liú)
Excess[161]	發生 (fā shēng)	赫曦 (hè xī)	敦阜 (dūn fù)	堅成 (jiān chéng)	流衍 (liú yǎn)

Ji of even qi years

Year of	Even Wood	Even Fire	Even Earth	Even Metal	Even Water
I do not understand these lines, but they seem important, so I am including them as they are	木德周行 (mù dé zhōu xíng) 陽舒陰布 (yáng shū yīn bù)	正陽而治 (zhèng yáng ér zhì) 德施周普 (dé shī zhōu pǔ)	氣協天休 (qì xié tiān xiū) 德流四政 (dé liú sì zhèng)	收而不爭 (shōu ér bù zhēng) 殺而無犯 (shā ér wú fàn)	藏而勿害 (cáng ér wù hài) 洽而普下 (zhì ér shàn xià)
5 Transformations	宣平 (xuān píng)	均衡 (jūn héng)	齊脩 (qí xiū)	宣明 (xuān míng)	咸整 (xián zhěng)
Qi	Straight[162]	High	Even	Clean	Bright
Nature	Follow 隨 (suí)	Speedy 速 (sù)	Submissive 順 (shùn)	Rigid 剛 (gāng)	Lower 下 (xià)
Use/Function	Flex Extend	Burn Scorch	High Low	Scatter Drop	Irrigate Flood[163]
Transformation	Rise Prosper	Flourish Luxuriate	Plump Fill	Harden Restrain	Congeal Harden
Type	Grass and trees	Fire	Earth	Metal	Water
Governance	Release Disperse	Brighten Shine	Calm Quiet	Force Silence	Flow[164] Emanate[165]
Climate	Warm moderate	Hot[166] Summerheat	Humidify[167] Steam	Clear Cut	Freeze Silence

Year of	Even Wood	Even Fire	Even Earth	Even Metal	Even Water
Command[168]	Wind	Heat	Damp	Dry	Cold
Zang	Liver	Heart	Spleen	Lung	Kidney
Zang fears ~	Cool[169]	Cold	Wind	Heat	Damp
Governs	Eyes	Tongue	Mouth	Nose	Urethra/Anus
Grain	Hemp	Wheat	Millet	Rice	Bean
Fruit	Plum	Apricot	Jujube	Peach	Chestnut
Solid? Fruit 實 (shí)[170]	Core 核 (hé)	Fibers 絡 (luò)	Flesh 肉 (ròu)	Shell 殼 (ké)	Soggy? Juice? 濡 (rú)
Reflects	Spring	Summer	Longsummer	Autumn	Winter
Creature	Furry	Feathered	Naked	Shelled	Scaly
Livestock	Dog	Horse	Ox	Chicken	Pig
Color	Blue-gray	Scarlet-red	Yellow	White	Black
Nourish	Sinews	Blood	Flesh	Skin/Body hair	Bone/Marrow
Condition	*Tenesmus*[171] *Propping Fullness*[172]	*Eye Twitch*[173] *Clonic Convulsion*[174]	*Glomus*[175]	*Cough*[176]	*Reversal*[177]
Flavor	Sour	Bitter	Sweet	Spicy	Salty
Sound	Mi 角 (jiǎo)	So 徵 (zhēng)	Do 宮 (gōng)	Re 商 (shāng)	La 羽 (yǔ)
Substance	Center hard	Vessel	Surface	Exterior hard	Soggy
Number	8	7	5	9	6

General guidelines for even qi

Qi Bo says, "Therefore generate/birth and do not kill, grow and do not punish, transform and do not limit, harvest and do not harm, store/hide and do not repress. This is known as even qi." He continues in a similar vein, detailing the characteristics of the years when the five elements are insufficient and/or excess. It is very poetic, quite long, and rather incomprehensible, though it seems like the insufficient years include aspects of their own element combined with the element that controls it (e.g. the Year of Insufficient Wood has Liver as its Zang, but jujube and plum as its fruit, sour and acrid as its flavor, white and blue-gray as its color, etc.). There is substantially more here than my basic charts can encompass. I will distill only the parts which seem most clinically relevant.

Clinically relevant aspects of insufficient years

Insufficient year of	Qi movement	Conditions
Wood	Restrained 斂 (liǎn)	*Limb(s) Atrophy* 肢痿 (zhī wěi) *Carbuncle Swelling* 癰腫 (yōng zhǒng) *Ulcers/Sores* 瘡瘍 (chuāng yáng)
Fire	Depressed 鬱 (yù)	*Dementia* 昏惑 (hūn huò) *Sadness* 悲 (bēi) *Forgetfulness* 忘 (wàng)
Earth	Scattered 散 (sàn)	*Food Stagnation* 留 (liú) *Fullness* 滿 (mǎn) *Glomus* 否 (pǐ) *Congestion* 塞 (sāi) *Lienteric Diarrhea* 飱泄 (sūn xiè)

Metal	Flight 揚 (yáng)	*Sneezing* 嚏 (tì) *Cough* 欬 (ké) *Nasal Congestion* 軌 (qiú) *Nosebleed* 衄 (nù)
Water	Stagnation 滯 (zhì)	*Atrophy Reversal* 痿厥 (wěi jué) *Hard Stools* 堅下 (jiān xià) *Urine Retention/Blockage* 癃閉 (lóng bì)

Effect of weather and geography on climate

Then the Emperor asks, "Sky is not sufficient in the west and north, left [is] cold and right [is] cool; land is not full in the east and south, right [is] hot and left [is] warm; why is this?"

Qi Bo answers, "This is due to the yin and yang of (qì) 氣 "weather," the higher and lower of (lǐ) 理 "geography," and the difference of (tài) 太 "greater" and (shào) 少 "lesser." East and south are yang, whose jīng-essence descends to the lower, therefore right is hot and left is warm. West and north are yin, whose jīng-essence is offered to the higher, therefore left is cold and right is cool. Therefore land has differing elevations, weather has differing temperatures. At high elevations, the weather is cold; at low elevations, the weather is hot. Therefore [those] accustomed to cold and cool [experience] *Distension*, [those] accustomed to] warm and hot [experience] *Carbuncles*; if purged, *Distension* occurs, and if sweat-induced, *Carbuncles* occur. This is the opening and closing of the interstices, also known as the difference of greater and lesser."

Lifespans and geography

The Emperor asks about lifespans. Qi Bo explains, "The person who honors yin essence lives long; the person whose yang essence descends dies young."

The Emperor asks about treatment. Qi Bo answers, "Scatter and make northwest qi cold. Gather and warm southeast qi. This is known as different treatment for the same disease." He elaborates on this for a few lines.

The next paragraph appears to be about geography, specifically altitude and how it affects the qi of lifespans. Then the Emperor asks about weather and how it controls qi [in people]. Qi Bo answers in detail.

Chronobiological rhythms of fertility and healing

The Emperor then asks about the chronobiological rhythms of fertility and healing. Qi Bo answers, "The six qì and five categories [of creatures] have a controlling cycle. When it matches, abundance ensues. When it differs, decline ensues. This is the Way of heaven and earth, the normal [rhythm] of generation and transformation." He goes through the fertility/infertility of furry, feathered, shelled, naked, and scaly animals based on which of the six channels (Jueyin, Shaoyin, Taiyin, Shaoyang, Yangming, Taiyang) are in charge of the heavenly stem or earthly branch position, and concludes, "Thus it is said, '[If one does] not know the addition of years, the sameness and difference of qi, [one] may not speak of generation and transformation.'"

The Emperor says, "When qi begins, generation and transformation happen. When qi scatters, there is form. When qi spreads, there is flourishing and reproduction. When qi ends, things change. However, the richness of the five flavors creates different thicknesses in generation and transformation, different amounts of maturity, different endings and beginnings. Why is this?"

Qi Bo says, "The qi of land controls it."

Land qi and flavors/colors of grain

在泉 (zài quán)*	Shaoyang	Yangming	Taiyang
~ toxin does not generate	Cold	Damp	Heat
Flavor	Spicy	Sour (qi damp)	Bitter
Treated by	Bitter, sour	Spicy, bitter, sweet	Bland, salty
Grain	Blue-gray, cinnabar	Cinnabar, plain	Golden-yellow, black

There is one line here about salty guarding the transformation of (chún) 淳 "pure," which is a character that has something to do with the pure flavor of wine, and spicy transforming concentrated qi to treat all of the above.

Basic herbology treatment principles

The final paragraph contains a lot of treatment principles that we still abide by today. To tonify above and below, follow the flow. To treat above and below, counter the flow. Those who can withstand toxins, give heavy [flavored] herbs. Those who cannot withstand toxins, give light herbs. If the qi is reversed, treat disease above from below, treat disease below from above, treat disease in the center from the sides. To treat cold using heat, warm and move. To treat heat using cold, cool and move. To treat warm using cool, chill and move. To treat cool using warm, heat and move. Thus, [the six techniques of] reducing, shaving, vomiting, draining, tonifying, and sedating may be used to treat chronic and new [diseases] alike. Formulas may be large or small, toxic or non-toxic. When treating, use very toxic herbs until the disease is 6/10ths better; regular toxic herbs, 7/10ths; slightly toxic herbs, 8/10ths; non-toxic herbs, 9/10ths. Dietary modifications involving grains, meats, fruits, and vegetables can be used until the condition is entirely gone, but do not overdo these, lest the upright qi be harmed. If [the

---

* See Appendix B for complete definition

condition is] not completely resolved, repeat, but be aware of the year and Solar Terms so as not to chop down the harmony of heaven, making excess more abundant or deficiency more deficient, creating catastrophe and shortening human life.

Emaciation and recovery

The Emperor asks one more question about (jí) 瘠 *Emaciation* after long illness. I am not entirely sure of Qi Bo's answer, but he seems to be saying, this is an excellent question, it is to be expected, and if you await the right season, carefully guarding the qi (Solar Term?), it is possible to nourish and harmonize a recovery.

Big Discussion on the Six Origins' Proper Records

六元正紀大論

(liù yuán zhèng jì dà lùn)

Chapter 71, Big Discussion on the Six Origins' Proper Records, details the governance of each of the six climatic factors, defines the first half of the year as belonging to (tiān qì) 天氣 "sky qi" or weather qi and the second half of the year as belonging to (dì qì) 地氣 "land qi" or geographic qi, and then goes into herbal treatment principles by five evolutive phase years. Then it describes the changes in weather abroad versus illness within the body depending on the five evolutive phase years' excess or insufficiency. The changes of the six climatic factors are tracked by arrival, transformation, governance, command, and function. General treatment principles for hot and cold herbs to release exterior or attack interior are explained at the end of the chapter.

There are some disease signs and symptoms that show up in this very long chapter, but they are sparse and intertwined with weather imagery and unfamiliar terminology, much of it very poetic. These chapters are clearly written by a different author from the rest of the book. The only paragraph that seems to consist entirely of symptoms occurs near the end:

Commonalities of disease (bìng zhī cháng) 病之常

Arrival of	Section 1	Section 2	Section 3	Section 4
Jueyin	*Tenesmus* 裡急 (lǐ jí)	*Armpit Pain* 支痛 (zhī tòng)	*Gnarled Cramps* 緛戾 (ruǎn lì)	*Rib Pain* 脇痛 (xié tòng) *Retching Diarrhea* 嘔泄 (ǒu xiè)
Shaoyin	*Lip Ulcers* 瘍胗 (yáng zhēn) *Body Hot* 身熱 (shēn rè)	*Shock-induced Disorientation* 驚惑 (jīng huò) *Aversion to Cold* 惡寒 (wù hán) *Trembling* 戰慄 (zhàn lì) *Delirium* 譫妄 (zhān wàng)	*Sadness-induced Delirium* 悲妄 (bēi wàng) *Epistaxis* 衄衊 (nù miè)	*Babbling* 語 (yǔ) *Laughter* 笑 (xiào)
Taiyin	*Accumulation Rheum* 積飲 (jī yǐn) *Glomus* 否 (pǐ) *Separation* 隔 (gé)	*Amassment* 蓄 (xù) *Fullness* 滿 (mǎn)	*Middle Fullness* 中滿 (zhōng mǎn) *Sudden Chaos* 霍亂 (huò luàn) *Vomiting/ Diarrhea* 吐下 (tù xià)	*Bilateral Foot Edema* 重胕腫 (chóng fù zhǒng)

Shaoyang	*Sneezing* 嚏 (tì) *Retching* 嘔 (ǒu) *Sores* 瘡 (chuāng) *Ulcers* 瘍 (yáng)	*Shock* 驚 (jīng) *Restlessness* 躁 (zào) *Blurry Vision/ Taste* 瞀昧 (mào wèi) *Violent Diseases* 暴病 (bào bìng)	*Throat Impediment* 喉痹 (hóu bì) *Tinnitus* 耳鳴 (ěr míng) *Reflux* 嘔涌 (ǒu yǒng)	*Violent Diarrhea* 暴注 (bào zhù) *Eye Twitch* 瞤 (rún) *Clonic Convulsion* 瘛 (chì) *Sudden Death* 暴死 (bào sǐ)
Yangming	*Floating Emptiness* 浮虛 (fú xū)	*Nasal Congestion* 䶌 (qiú) *Sacrum, Genital, Buttock, Knee, Hip, Calf, Shin and Leg Disease* 尻陰股膝髀 腨䯒足病 (kāo yīn gǔ xī bì chuǎn héng zú bìng)	*Chapped Skin* 皴揭 (cūn jiē)	*Nasal Congestion* 䶌 (qiú) *Sneezing* 嚏 (tì)
Taiyang	*Difficulty Flexing/ Extending* 屈伸不利 (qū shēn bú lì)	*Low Back Pain* 腰痛 (yāo tòng)	*Night Sweats* 寢汗 (qǐn hàn) *Convulsions* 痙 (jìng)	*Incontinence* 流泄禁止 (liú xiè jìn zhǐ)

This paragraph begins, "Jueyin Arrival is *Tenesmus*. Shaoyin Arrival is *Lip Ulcers*..." I am not sure why the text does not list all the symptoms for Jueyin first, then Shaoyin, Taiyin, and so on, but I have preserved the sequence, just in case it is significant.

Symptoms of Cold and Heat Arrival

Cold Arrival (hán zhì) 寒至: pathogenic Cold arrives during cold weather	*Hard Glomus* 堅否 (jiān pǐ) *Abdominal Fullness* 腹滿 (fù mǎn) *Painful Urgent Diarrhea* 痛急下利 (tòng jí xià lì)
Heat Arrival (rè zhì) 熱至: pathogenic Heat arrives during hot weather	*Body Hot* 身熱 (shēn rè) *Vomiting/Diarrhea* 吐下 (tù xià) *Sudden Chaos* 霍亂 (huò luàn) *Carbuncles, Abscesses, Sores, Ulcers* 癰疽瘡瘍 (yōng jū chuāng yáng) *Malaise with Dizziness* 瞀鬱 (mào yù) *Copious Watery Diarrhea* 注下 (zhù xià) *Eye Twitch* 瞤 (rún) *Clonic Convulsion* 瘛 (chì) *Swelling/Distension* 腫脹 (zhǒng zhàng) *Retching* 嘔 (ǒu) *Nasal Congestion with Epistaxis* 鼽衄 (qiú nǜ) *Headache* 頭痛 (tóu tòng) *Bony Joint Derangement* 骨節變 (gǔ jié biàn) *Myalgia* 肉痛 (ròu tòng) *Blood Upwelling* 血溢 (xiě yì) *Bloody Diarrhea* 血泄 (xiě xiè) *Painful Urine Retention* 淋閟 (lín bì)

According to Qi Bo, both Cold and Heat Arrival can be treated by "that which triumphs over" it.

Detoxing during pregnancy

The Emperor then asks about pregnant women with toxins. Qi Bo answers that treatment is possible "without damage" ...to the mother or the baby? He does not specify. He goes on to say, "*Great Accumulations* (dà jī) 大積 and *Great Gatherings* (dà jù) 大聚 may be treated. Stop after [the condition] is more than half recovered; the overtreated die." Again, he does not specify if the patient or the fetus dies, but I think this general concept can be stretched to include non-pregnant patients with really bad food stagnation or other abdominal lumps (i.e. impacted colon): once the condition begins to clear, we need only help it gather momentum to recover more than 50 percent, at which point treatment may stop and healing will continue on its own.

Discussion on Pricking Methods

刺法論

(cì fǎ lùn)

Chapter 72, Discussion on Pricking Methods, contains some actual point prescriptions.

Point prescriptions for freeing constrained ascending qi

"When **element** wishes to rise and is constrained, one should needle **point**:"	
Wood	Foot Jueyin jǐng-well (Liver 1)
Fire	Bāo Luò yíng-spring (Pericardium 8)
Earth	Foot Taiyin shū-stream (Spleen 3)
Metal	Hand Taiyin jīng-river (Lung 8)
Water	Foot Shaoyin hé-sea (Kidney 10)

---

*   The text of Chapters 72 and 73, originally lost, was allegedly written by 劉溫舒 (Liú Wēnshū) of the Song Dynasty (ca. 1098). Only the titles were listed in the 王冰 (Wáng Bīng) edition (ca. 672), and they are not included in Paul Unschuld's annotated translation.

Point prescriptions for preventing the suffocation of descending qi

Wood	Hand Taiyin exit (Lu11), Hand Yangming entry (LI1)
Fire	Foot Shaoyin exit (K22), Foot Taiyang entry (UB1)
Earth	Foot Jueyin exit (Lv14), Foot Shaoyang entry (GB1)
Metal	Pericardium exit (P8), Hand Shaoyang entry (SJ1)
Water	Foot Taiyin exit (Sp21), Foot Yangming entry (St1)

Chronobiological point prescriptions

I am not sure what the next section's diagnostic indications are. I think they have something to do with preventing imbalances in the chronobiological tendencies of previous chapters.

Running late

~ (fù bù) 復布	~ (wèi dé qiān zhèng) 未得遷正	Drain [point]
Taiyang	Jueyin	Foot Jueyin flow (Lv2)
Jueyin	Shaoyin	Pericardium flow (P8)
Shaoyin	Taiyin	Foot Taiyin flow (Sp2)
Taiyin	Shaoyang	Hand Shaoyang flow (SJ2)
Shaoyang	Yangming	Hand Taiyin flow (Lu10)
Yangming	Taiyang	Foot Shaoyin flow (K2)

That chart was for running late (i.e. Jueyin not arriving at the appropriate time due to Taiyang lingering). The next chart is for running early (i.e. Jueyin lingering and causing Wood transformation issues in the weather). However, I do not know the meaning of the terms fù bù, wèi dé qiān zhèng, or bú tuì wèi.

Running early

Years	~ (bú tuì wèi) 不退位	~ dominates the weather	Needle [point]
巳亥 (sì hài)	Jueyin	Wind/Wood	Foot Jueyin entry (Lv1)
子午 (zǐ wǔ)	Shaoyin	Heat/Fire	Hand Jueyin entry (P1)
丑未 (chǒu wèi)	Taiyin	Damp/Rain	Foot Taiyin entry (Sp1)
寅申 (yín shēn)	Shaoyang	Heat/Fire	Hand Shaoyang entry (SJ1)
卯酉 (mǎo yǒu)	Yangming	Metal/Dryness	Hand Taiyin entry (Lu1)
辰戌 (chén xū)	Taiyang	Cold/Water	Foot Shaoyin entry (K1)

Post-treatment instructions for aftercare

Now the chapter gets really complicated. They go on to discuss three-year predictions of epidemics due to weather resonances. What I find interesting about this section are the instructions for aftercare. For example, for all chronic Kidney conditions, after the acupuncture (UB23 followed by three days of Sp3), [the patient should] face south during the hour of 03:00-05:00 寅 (yín), hold the breath and swallow qi as if swallowing an extremely hard object seven times. After the acupuncture for (bǐng yín) 丙寅 years (UB15 followed by five days of K10), the patient should be cautious against great joy or desires within for seven days. After the acupuncture for (gēng chén) 庚辰 years (UB18 followed by three days of Lu8), the patient should avoid great anger for seven days. After the acupuncture for (rèn wǔ) 壬午 years (UB20 followed by three days of Lv14), the patient should avoid getting very drunk, singing, overeating, or eating overly sour or raw foods, and it is best to keep the diet bland for seven days. After the acupuncture for (wù shēn) 戊申 years (UB13), the patient should avoid great sadness for seven days.

Preventing the spread of epidemic diseases

The Emperor then asks about contagion, and how one might attain non-spreading of the five epidemic diseases. Qi Bo answers with the famous and oft-quoted,

正氣存內, 邪不可干。

(zhèng qì cún nèi, xié bù kě gān)

If there is upright qi within, pathogens cannot interfere.* He describes a visualization for entering the sick room. "Imagine the heart as the sun... Imagine blue-green qi exuding from the liver, traveling left on the east to become a forest of trees. Then imagine white qi exuding from the lung, traveling right on the west to become weapons and armor. Then imagine red qi exuding from the heart, traveling south above to become the brightness of flames. Then imagine black qi exuding from the kidney, traveling north below to become water. Then imagine yellow qi exuding from the spleen, preserved in the center as earth. With these five qi protecting you, then imagine light above the head like that of the Big Dipper, then [you] may enter the sick room."

He also offers three alternate methods for warding off epidemic disease:

1. Induce vomiting before dawn on the Solar Term (chūn fēn) 春分 "Spring Equinox"

2. Induce sweating through three herbal baths after the Solar Term (yǔ shuǐ) 雨水 "Rain Water"

3. Small golden pellet formula: cinnabar 2 liǎng, water-ground realgar 1 liǎng, leaf orpiment 1 liǎng, purple gold 1 liǎng. Fire with 20 jīn for 7 days, let cool for 7 days, bury in the ground for 7 days, grind for 3 days into a fine powder, make honey balls the size of sycamore seeds, take 1 pellet with ice water facing east on inhalation. After 10 pellets, no epidemic disease can interfere

---

*   「正氣存內, 邪不可干。」 (zhèng qì cún nèi, xié bù kě gān).

Point prescriptions for constitutional deficiencies exacerbated by chronobiology

The final paragraph of this chapter covers a number of point prescriptions for constitutional deficiencies exacerbated by deficiencies in heaven and earth. I am a little skeptical about their usefulness, since the first half mentions possession by zombies in the colors of the five elements and the second half seems to be directly plagiarized from Chapter 8, but here they are:

Disease	Etiology[178]	Needle
Jueyin off guard, Liver deficient	(hún) 魂 "Ethereal soul" wanders upward	Foot Shaoyang's passage (GB40) and Liver shū (UB18)
Heart deficient with imperial/ministerial fire off guard, fire insufficient	Black zombie attacks	Hand Shaoyang's passage (SJ4) and Heart shū (UB15)
Spleen disease with Taiyin offguard, earth insufficient	Green zombie attacks	Foot Yangming's passage (St42) and Spleen shū (UB20)
Lung disease with Yangming offguard, metal insufficient	Red zombie attacks	Hand Yangming's passage (LI4) and Lung shū (UB13)
Kidney disease with Taiyang offguard, water insufficient year[179]	Yellow zombie sucks shén-spirit and hún-ethereal soul	Foot Taiyang's passage (UB64) and Foot Shaoyang shū (UB19)

Organ	Official of ~之官 (zhī guān)	Duties (~ are exuded by it) ~出焉 (chū yān)	May needle
Heart	Emperor 君主 (jūn zhǔ)	Spirit and brightness 神明 (shén míng)	Hand Shaoyin yuán-source (H7)

Lung	Minister 相傅 (xiāng fù)	Governance and regularity* 治節 (zhì jié)	Hand Taiyin yuán-source (Lu9)
Liver	General 將軍 (jiāng jūn)	Strategy and planning 謀慮 (móu lǜ)	Foot Jueyin yuán-source (Lv3)
Gallbladder	Justice 中正 (zhōng zhèng)	Judgment and decisions 決斷 (jué duàn)	Foot Shaoyang yuán-source (GB40)
Pericardium[180]	Jester 臣使 (chén shǐ)	Joy and music 喜樂 (xǐ yuè)	Pericardium luò-collateral's flow point (P8?)
Spleen	Discusser 諫議 (jiàn yì)	Knowing the big picture 知周 (zhī zhōu)	Spleen yuán-source (Sp3)
Stomach	Granary 倉廩 (cāng lǐn)	5 flavors 五味 (wǔ wèi)	Stomach yuán-source (St42)
Large Intestine	Transport 傳道 (chuán dào)	Change and transformation 變化 (biàn huà)	Large Intestine yuán-source (LI4)
Small Intestine	Sorter 受盛 (shòu shèng)	Transforming substance 化物 (huà wù)	Small Intestine yuán-source (SI3)
Kidney	Strengthener 做強 (zuò qiáng)	Talent and agility 伎巧 (jì qiǎo)	Kidney yuán-source (K3)
Sānjiao	Irrigation 決瀆 (jué dú)	Waterways 水道 (shuǐ dào)	Sānjiao yuán-source (SJ4)

---

* 節 (jié): solar terms, regularity, seasonal nodes, joints, holidays, moderation, governance and regulation... I am guessing Lung is in charge of interfacing between the body and the 24 Solar Terms, since it interacts most directly with seasonal weather changes. Giovanni Maciocia's book <u>The Foundations of Chinese Medicine</u> (volume 3, p.132) goes with regulation. Although, if we want the format to match, perhaps (zhì jié) 治節 means "governance/organization and moderation/abnegation"...that fits with metal.

Bladder	Wetlands 州都 (zhōu dū)	Stores fluids, qi transformation [required] for exudation 「津液藏焉, 氣化則能出矣」 (jīn yè cáng yān, qì huà zé néng chū yǐ)	Bladder yuán-source (UB64)

The chapter ends with some remarks about nourishing (zhēn) 真 the "true" which sounds more Daoist than all previous passages, even Chapter 1.

Discussion on Root Diseases

本病論

(běn bìng lùn)

The source of Chapter 73, Discussion on Root Diseases, is even more murky than that of Chapter 72. I am not sure if Liú actually wrote the text I am reading, or if he copied it from somewhere. The text contains passages alluding to shamanic beliefs that conflict with the tone of the rest of the book. However, the very last paragraph has a few interesting details about activities which harm the shén-spirit and I find these valuable.

Consequences of certain emotions/activities

Actions	Harms	Actions	~ exudes sweat
Worry, longing, thinking, anticipation	Heart	Shock robs jing-essence	Heart
Drinking, eating, overexertion	Spleen	Overeating Sex while drunk or overfull	Stomach Spleen
Prolonged sitting in damp place, exerting force in water	Kidney		
Rage or anger, qi counterflows upward and does not descend	Liver	Sprinting in fear	Liver

This is not to say the passages before this last paragraph are not valuable; there are lots of clusters of symptoms describing various patterns but I find them confusingly linked to states calculated from the heavenly branches and earthly stems. For example, there are definitions to terms such as (qì jiāo) 氣交 "Qi Exchange" and (shī shǒu) 失守 "Lose Guard."

Big Discussion on the Essentials of Ultimate Truth

至真要大論

(zhì zhēn yào dà lùn)

Chapter 74, Big Discussion on the Essentials of Ultimate Truth, is a really long chapter which covers how the six climatic factors affect the weather, condition pathogenesis, pulse diagnosis, and herbal treatment (mostly in terms of the five flavors). There are also details on the signs and symptoms arising from (shèng) 勝 *Triumph* and (fù) 復 *Retaliation*, treatment principles, formula composition, root and branch, prognosis, treatment planning, and pathogenesis. I have read the famous (bìng jī shí jiuˇ tiáo) 病機十九條 "19 Lines of Pathogenesis" before, but not the yin and yang functions of the five flavors and the applications of treatment principles that come after this.

The effect of the six climatic factors on weather

Transformation 化 (huà)	Jueyin 厥陰	Shaoyin 少陰	Taiyin 太陰	Shaoyang 少陽	Yangming 陽明	Taiyang 太陽
First half of year 司天 (sī tiān)	Wind (fēng) 風	Heat (rè) 熱	Damp (shī) 濕	Fire (huǒ) 火	Dry (zào) 燥	Cold (hán) 寒
Second half of year 在泉 (zài quán)*	Sour (suān) 酸	Bitter (kǔ) 苦	Sweet (gān) 甘	Bitter (kǔ) 苦	Spicy (xīn) 辛	Salty (xián) 鹹
Dominant qi 司氣 (sī qì)	Blue-gray (cāng) 蒼	None[181]	Golden-yellow (jīn) 黅	Cinnabar (dān) 丹	Plain (sù) 素	Dark (xuán) 玄
Between qi 間氣 (jiān qì)	Move (dòng) 動	Scorch[182] (zhuó) 灼	Soften (róu) 柔	Brighten (míng) 明	Clear (qīng) 清	Hide (cáng) 藏

The next section contains a few gems of wisdom worth quoting.

On pathogenesis

謹候氣宜, 無失病機

(jǐn hòu qì yí, wú shī bìng jī)

Observe the climatic factors closely, and [you shall] not miss
the pathogenesis.

On authentic herbs

司歲備物

(sī suì bèi wù)

Prepare [herbal] substances in dominant years,

則無遺主

(zé wú yí zhǔ)

then [you shall] not lose the chief [qualities].

---

*   See Appendix B for complete definition

How to observe and regulate yin and yang via pulses

Even pulse	Carotid and radial pulse match in size, like pulling ropes				
Second half of year	Shaoyin	Jueyin	Taiyin	3 yins	3 yins in first half of year
Does not match	radial pulse	right pulse	left pulse	chǐ-cubit pulse	cùn-inch pulse

Skipping over the symptoms that are tangled with weather forecasting, we come to basic formula composition guidelines.

Basic formula composition: flavors/actions for (zài quán) 在泉

(qì zài quán) 氣在泉 "Qi at the [water] spring," i.e. dominant qi of second half of year						
Dominant	Wind	Heat	Damp	Fire	Dry	Cold
Treat with	spicy cool	salty cold	bitter hot	salty cold	bitter warm	sweet hot
Envoy	bitter	sweet bitter	sour bland	bitter spicy	sweet spicy	bitter spicy
Action	relax	astringe	dry	astringe	descend	astringe
Flavor	with sweet	with sour	with bitter	with sour	with bitter	with sour
Action	scatter	release	drain	release		drain
Flavor	with spicy	with bitter	with bland	with bitter		with salty

293

Basic formula composition: flavors/actions for (sī tiān) 司天

(sī tiān zhī qì) 司天之氣 "Qi which commands the sky," i.e. dominant qi of first half of year

Dominant	Wind	Heat	Damp[183]	Fire	Dry	Cold
Balance with	spicy cool	salty cold	bitter hot	sour cold[184]	bitter warm	spicy hot
Envoy	bitter sweet	bitter sweet	sour spicy	bitter sweet	sour spicy	sweet bitter
Action	slow	astringe	dry drain	astringe	descend	drain
Flavor	with sweet	with sour	with bitter with bland	with sour	with bitter	with salty

Basic formula composition: flavors/actions for pathogenic qi in second half of year

(xié qì fǎn shèng) 邪氣反勝 "Pathogenic qi overcomes" [dominant qi] in second half of year

Dominant	Wind	Heat	Damp	Fire	Dry[185]	Cold
Pathogenic	cool	cold	heat	cold	heat	heat
Treat with	sour warm	sweet hot	bitter cold[186]	sweet hot	neutral cold	salty cold
Envoy	bitter sweet	bitter spicy	salty sweet	bitter spicy	bitter sweet	sweet spicy
Balance	with spicy	with salty	with bitter	with salty	with sour	with bitter

Basic formula composition: flavors/actions for pathogenic qi in first half of year

(xié qì fǎn shèng) 邪氣反勝 "Pathogenic qi overcomes" [dominant qi] in first half of year						
Dominant	Wind	Heat	Damp	Fire	Dry	Cold
Pathogenic	cool	cold	hot	cold	heat	heat
Treat with	sour warm	sweet warm	bitter cold	sweet hot	spicy cold	salty cold[187]
Envoy	sweet bitter	bitter sour spicy	bitter sour	bitter spicy	bitter sweet	bitter spicy

Basic formula composition: flavors/actions for (shèng) 勝 *Triumph* of 6 climatic factors

Triumph of	Jueyin	Shaoyin	Taiyin	Shaoyang	Yangming	Taiyang
Treat with	sweet cool	spicy cold	salty hot	spicy cold	sour warm	sweet hot
Envoy	bitter spicy	bitter salty	spicy sweet	sweet salty	spicy sweet	spicy sour
Drain with	sour	sweet	bitter	sweet	bitter	salty

Basic formula composition: flavors/actions for (fù) 復 *Retaliations* of 6 climatic factors

Retaliation of	Jueyin	Shaoyin[188]	Taiyin	Shaoyang	Yangming	Taiyang
Treat with	sour cold	salty cold	bitter hot	salty chill	spicy warm	salty hot
Envoy	sweet spicy	bitter spicy	sour spicy	bitter spicy	bitter sweet	sweet spicy
Action	drain with	drain with	drain with	soften with	drain with	harden with
Flavor	sour	sweet	bitter	salty	bitter	bitter
~ with	slow	astringe release soften	dry drain	astringe release	descend tonify	
Flavor	sweet	sour spicy bitter salty	[bitter]	sour spicy bitter[189]	bitter sour	

General Treatment Principles

治諸勝復,
(zhì zhū shèng fù,)
To treat all *Triumphs* and *Retaliations*,

寒者熱之, 熱者寒之,
(hán zhě rè zhī, rè zhě hán zhī,)
heat what is cold, chill what is hot,

溫者清之, 清者溫之,
(wēn zhě qīng zhī, qīng zhě wēn zhī,)
warm what is cool, cool what is warm,

散者收之, 抑者散之,
(sàn zhě shōu zhī, yì zhě sàn zhī,)
astringe what is scattered, disperse what is constrained,

燥者潤之, 急者緩之

(zào zhě rùn zhī, jí zhě huǎn zhī)

moisten what is dry, slow/ease what is urgent,

堅者耎之, 脆者堅之

(jiān zhě ruǎn zhī, cuì zhě jiān zhī)

soften what is hard, harden what is brittle,

衰者補之, 強者寫之

(shuāi zhě bǔ zhī, jiàng zhě xiè zhī)

tonify what is frail, drain what is stiff,

各安其氣, 必清必靜

(gè ān qí qì, bì qīng bì jìng)

calm each type of qi, require clarity and quietude,

則病氣衰去, 歸其所宗

(zé bìng qì shuāi qù, guī qí suǒ zōng)

then disease qi weakens and goes back to its source.

St25 as the Equator of the Body and how it relates to *Triumph* and *Retaliation*

Upper body is governed by sky qi, i.e. the first half of the year. Lower body is governed by land qi, i.e. the second half of the year, also known as (mìng qì) 命氣 "life qi." The midline is (tiān shū) 天樞 "Sky Pivot" St25. If both *Triumph* and *Retaliation* disease states occur, always name it by the retaliation qi. The Beginning to Third Qi Cycle is governed by sky qi; the fourth to End Qi Cycle is governed by land qi. If there is *Triumph* (in the first to third Qi Cycle), then there will be *Retaliation* (in the fourth to sixth Qi Cycle).

There are also cases where the (kè qì) 客氣 "guest qi" triumphs but the (zhǔ qì) 主氣 "master qi" progresses as usual, where *Retaliation* does not occur. Guest qi is an alternate name for the six climatic factors' qi. Master qi refers to the six 步 (bù) "steps" of the four seasons controlled by between qi.

More herbal treatment principles

There is a huge list of symptoms, followed by these herbal treatment principles: Restrain the high. Raise the low. Fracture excess. Mend insufficiency. Envoy with [what is] beneficial. Harmonize with [what is] appropriate. Must calm the host and guest. Moderate the cold and hot. Counter that which is the same (i.e. use cold herbs to counter hot host, hot guest). Follow that which is different.

Master	Wood	Fire	Earth	Metal	Water
Drain	Sour	Sweet	Bitter	Spicy	Salty
Tonify	Spicy	Salty	Sweet	Sour	Bitter

Guest	Jueyin	Shaoyin	Taiyin	Shaoyang	Yangming	Taiyang
Tonify	Spicy	Salty	Sweet	Salty	Sour	Bitter
Drain	Sour	Sweet	Bitter	Sweet	Spicy	Salty
Flavor	Sweet	Salty	Sweet	Salty	Bitter	Bitter
Action	Relax	Astringe	Relax	Soften	Drain	Harden

In addition, for Taiyang it is advised to use spicy to moisten, open and release the interstices, to improve the throughput of qi and body fluids.

Number of herbs per formula according to *Dà Yào* 《大要》 <u>Big Essentials</u>

Emperor	1	2	2	2
Deputy	2	4	3	6
Combination	Odd	Even	Odd	Even

Additional tips on formula composition

Recent onset, use odds. Long-standing, use evens. Sweating, avoid odds. Descending, avoid evens. Tonifying or treating above, formulate slow. Tonifying or treating below, formulate urgent. Urgent means thick flavors; slow means thin flavors. Recent onset, use small formulas, down to 2 herbs. Long-standing [issue], use large formulas, up to 9 herbs.

Double Formula	Reverse Envoy
重方 (chóng fāng):	反佐 (fǎn zuǒ):
If an odd formula does not resolve the issue, then use an even formula	If an even formula does not resolve the issue, then reverse the envoy herb/s

病反其本, 得標之病,
(bìng fǎn qí běn, dé biāo zhī bìng)
If the disease arises not from the root, but from the branch,

治反其本, 得標之方。
(zhì fǎn qí běn, dé biāo zhī fāng.)
treat in reverse, against the root, to get the formula for the branch.

	Root	Branch	Middle
Shaoyang	X		
Taiyin	X		
Shaoyin	X	X	
Taiyang	X	X	
Yangming			X
Jueyin			X

19 Lines of Pathogenesis

	All	Belong to
1.	Wind, Falls, Vertigo	Liver
2.	Cold, Contraction, Pulling	Kidney
3.	Air, Huffing, Depression	Lung
4.	Damp, Swelling, Fullness	Spleen
5.	Heat, Vision distortion, Convulsions	Fire
6.	Pain, Itching, Ulcers	Heart
7.	Reversal, Constipation, Diarrhea	Below
8.	Atrophy, Panting, Retching	Above
9.	Shuddering, Chattering, as if losing one's mind	Fire
10.	Nape tension	Damp
11.	Counterflow rushing upward	Fire
12.	Distension, Abdomen enlargement	Heat
13.	Restlessness, Mania, Straying	Fire
14.	Violent rigidity	Wind
15.	Diseases with drum-like sounds	Heat
16.	Feet edema, Aching pain, Shock terror	Fire
17.	Turning, Opposition, Perversity, Fluids turbid	Heat
18.	Diseases with fluids clear and cool	Cold
19.	Retching, Vomiting acid, Sudden diarrhea, Bowel urgency	Heat

Formula size

	Small	Medium	Large
Emperor	1	1	1
Deputy	2	3	3
Envoy	0	5	9

Treatment principles

Disease	Treatment
Cold	Heat
Heat	Cold
Faint	Counterflow
Extreme	Following
Hard	Pare away
Guest (exterior pathogens)	Dispel
Taxation	Warm
Knotted	Scatter
Lingering	Attack
Dry	Soak
Urgent/Acute	Slow down/Relax
Scattered	Contract
Damaged	Warm
Sedentary	Move
Shock	Balance
Ascending	Descend
(mó) 摩 Scoured	Bathe
Thin	Arrest
Open	Release
Spread from interior to exterior	Regulate interior
Spread from exterior to interior	Treat the exterior
Interior to exterior but exterior signs severe	Regulate interior first, then treat the exterior
Exterior to interior but interior signs severe	Treat the exterior first, then regulate the interior
Internal and external diseases unrelated	Treat main disease
Cooling treatment generates Heat signs	Yin
Warming treatment generates Cold signs	Yang

Flavors: adding qi into the five Zang over time

Flavor	Sour	Bitter	Sweet	Spicy	Salty
Enters ~ first	Liver	Heart	Spleen	Lung	Kidney

Definitions of (jūn) 君 Emperor, (chén) 臣 Deputy, (shǐ) 使 Envoy

Emperor: for main condition	Deputy: envoy of Emperor	Assistant: obey Deputy

Qi Bo emphasizes here that Emperor, Deputy, and Envoy do NOT mean Superior, Common, and Inferior herbs.*

---

* 岐伯曰:「主病之謂君，佐君之謂臣，應臣之謂使，非上下三品之謂也。」
(zhǔ bìng zhī wèi jūn, zuǒ jūn zhī wèi chén, yìng chén zhī wèi shǐ, fēi shàng xià sān pǐn zhī wèi yě).

Discussion Illuminating Ultimate Teachings

著至教論

(zhù zhì jiào lùn)

Chapter 75, Discussion Illuminating Ultimate Teachings, departs from the question-and-answer with Qi Bo format and introduces a new character, Léi Gōng 雷公 "thunder male-honorific," who seems to be the Emperor's student.

The Emperor summons Lei Gong and asks, "Do you know the Way of medicine?"

Lei Gong answers humbly that he can recite and sort of understand some, but not really differentiate with clarity. He claims that his skills are enough to treat the masses but insufficient for treating the aristocracy.

The Emperor says, "Yes. This is all about the transportation and reflection of yin and yang, exterior and interior, up and down, male and female. Knowing astrology above, geography below, and human affairs in the middle, [you] will pass this medical knowledge to future generations, to the common people, as treasures."

Lei Gong says, "Please teach [me]."

The Emperor asks, "Have you heard of the pathophysiology of yin and yang?"

Lei Gong says, "No." So the Emperor begins telling him about yang. If three yang arrive simultaneously above, it will create (diān jí) 巔疾 *Vertex Disease*; below, it creates (lòu bìng) 漏病 *Leaking Disease*. If three yang merges with (jī) 積 *Accumulation* then there is (jīng) 驚 *Shock* with onset sudden as wind and thunder, the orifices are clogged, the esophagus is dry, and the trachea is congested. Combined with yin and there is no regularity ascending or descending, which creates (cháng pì) 腸癖 *Intestinal Blockage*.

The Emperor emphasizes how important it is to be able to differentiate yin from yang, to reflect the four seasons, and harmonize the five elements. Lei Gong (formally) requests again to be taught. I cannot tell from the Emperor's answer if he has agreed to teach him; he admonishes Lei Gong against confusion and unclear, undifferentiated learning.

Chapter 76

Discussion on Indications Following Countenance

示從容論

(shì cóng róng lùn)

Chapter 76, Discussion on Indications Following Countenance, contains two case studies that Lei Gong is confused about. The Emperor summons Lei Gong and asks him how his studies, technique, and memorization are progressing. Lei Gong says he has been reading the *Mài Jīng* 《脈經》 <u>Pulse Classic</u>. The Emperor encourages his student to ask questions.

Lei Gong's Case Study #1

Lei Gong says, "Liver deficiency, Kidney deficiency, [and] Spleen deficiency* all create (tǐ zhòng) 體重 *Body Heaviness* and (fán yuān) 煩冤 *Vexation Grievance*, to be treated by herbs or

---

* 「肝虛腎虛脾虛」 (gān xū shèn xū pí xū).

needles or moxibustion or biǎn stones. However, some cases are cured and some are not. [I] would like to hear this explained."

The Emperor explains that when Spleen floats deficiently like Lung, when Kidney floats slightly like Spleen, when Liver is tight deep and scattered like Kidney, these signs indicate that the practitioner created the mess, or (luàn) 亂 "chaos." Interestingly, the character for "chaos" is the same one as used for "revolution" in Chapter 2. The Emperor tells Lei Gong his question is elementary, like a child's question.

Lei Gong then gives a case example to illustrate his confusion. "A person with (tóu tòng) 頭痛 *Headache*, (jīn luán) 筋攣 *Sinew Cramps*, (gǔ zhòng) 骨重 *Bone Heaviness*, (qiè rán) 怯然 *Fearfulness*, (shǎo qì) 少氣 *Scant Qi*, (yuě) 噦 *Belching*, (yì) 噫 *Hiccups*, (fù mǎn) 腹滿 *Abdominal Fullness*, (shí jīng) 時驚 *Periodic Shock*, and (bú shì wò) 不時臥 *Irregular Sleep*, which Zang is expressing? The pulse is floating and wiry, hard as a stone. [I] do not know which of the three Zang this is."

The Emperor says, "[You] speak of (cóng róng) 從容 'following countenance.' Look to the Fu for the elderly, the channels for the young, the Zang for those in their prime. Floating and wiry indicates Kidney insufficiency. Deep and stone-hard indicates Kidney qi is inside. (qiè rán) 怯然 *Fearfulness* and (shǎo qì) 少氣 *Scant Qi* indicates the waterways [are] not flowing. (ké sòu) 欬嗽 *Cough* with (fán yuān) 煩冤 *Vexation Grievance* indicates Kidney qi counterflow."

Lei Gong's Case Study #2

Lei Gong then asks, "[I saw a] person with (sì zhī xiè duò) 四支 解憜 *Fatigue in Four Limbs*, (chuǎn) 喘 *Panting*, (ké) 欬 *Cough*, and (xiě xiè) 血泄 *Bloody Diarrhea*. I thought it was Lung damage; the pulse was floating, large, and tight. I did not have the confidence to treat; a lesser practitioner used biǎn stones, which created more bleeding. What is this?"

The Emperor explains that a floating, large deficient pulse indicates Spleen qi terminating outside, out beyond the Stomach which belongs to Yangming. When two fires cannot control three waters, the pulse become chaotic and disregulated. (sì zhī xiè duò) 四支解墮 *Fatigue in Four Limbs* indicates Spleen essence [is] not moving. (chuǎn) 喘 *Panting* and (ké) 欬 *Cough* indicate water qi in the Yangming. (xiě xiè) 血泄 *Bloody Diarrhea* indicates vessels contracting, leaving the blood nowhere to flow.

He says some more disparaging things to Lei Gong about how Lung damage is the wrong diagnosis. I like the Emperor better when he was learning from Qi Bo. He was eager and humble as a student; he is rather mean as the instructor.

Discussion on Five Neglectful Mistakes

疏五過論

(shū wǔ guò lùn)

In Chapter 77, Discussion on Five Neglectful Mistakes, the Emperor tells Lei Gong of five mistakes made by practitioners.

First the Emperor makes some exclamations about looking into the deep abyss and meeting floating clouds, which I hope are not pertinent, then he asks if Lei Gong has heard of (wǔ guò) 五過 "Five Mistakes" and (sì dé) 四 德 "Four Virtues."

Lei Gong makes obeisance and says, "Your vassal is young, ignorant, and confused, and has not heard of Five Mistakes and Four Virtues."

Five Mistakes

The Five Mistakes are diagnostic oversights.

- Mistake 1. Not asking whether the patient has been lowered in class after having been high-class, which creates an internally generated condition called (tuō yíng) 脫營 *Desertion of Nourishment*, and whether they have become poor after having been wealthy, which creates a condition called (shī jīng) 失精 *Loss of Essence*. The practitioner cannot find the cause of weight loss, qi deficiency, periodic shock, exhaustion of defensive and nutritive qi in the Zang nor the body.

- Mistake 2. Not asking about diet, lifestyle, and sudden emotions. (bào nù) 暴怒 *Violent Anger* harms yin; (bào xǐ) 暴喜 *Violent Joy* harms the yang. [This will cause] qi to ascend in *Reversal*, filling the vessels and messing up the body. If a foolish doctor does not know how to tonify or drain accordingly, the essence and aura will disconnect and pathogens may enter.

- Mistake 3. Assuming that pulse diagnosis is not important because one is not adept at it.

- Mistake 4. Coming back to Mistake 1, if one loses power after having been granted it, jīng-essence and shén-spirit will be harmed internally and manifest as defeat in the body. If one starts off wealthy and then becomes poor, even without pathogens the skin will dry and sinews will bend, creating (wěi bì) 痿躄 *Atrophy Lameness* and (luán) 攣 *Cramps*. The doctor must not be strict, must not move the shén-spirit unduly. The external will be fragile and soft; chaos will result in dysregulation. The condition cannot be shifted. Treatment will become impossible.

- Mistake 5. Diagnosis of (fēng) 風 *Wind* must include knowledge of ending and beginning, and sequence. Pulse reading and asking should be appropriate to gender...if the practitioner treats sloppily, the body falls apart, the four limbs cramp, and death is imminent. If the doctor cannot be clear, does not ask for the history of how this came to be, but only speaks of the predicted death date, this is also sloppy practice.

Required knowledge for treating like a sage

In conclusion, to treat as the sages did, one must know (tiān) 天 "weather/astrology" and (dì) 地 "land/geography," (yīn) 陰 and (yáng) 陽, (sì shí) 四時 "four seasons," (jīng jì) 經紀 "channels and records," five Zang, six Fu, female versus male, exterior versus interior, pricking versus moxibustion, (biǎn shí) 砭石 "bloodletting stones" versus (dú yào) 毒藥 "toxic herbs." One must also be clear about high versus low class, wealth versus poverty, age versus youth, courage versus timidity. Observe the components to know the root and onset of disease. The Way to treatment is to treasure qi within and follow the grain or intrinsic texture.* If attempts yield no results, the mistake is in exterior-interior. There are a few more sentences here but I think they are just emphasizing importance, not actually substantial in content.

The lost books from Chapter 46 (*Shàng Jīng* 《上經》 Upper Classic, *Xià Jīng* 《下經》 Lower Classic, *Kuí Duó* 《揆度》 Formulas and Pulses, *Qí Héng* 《奇恆》 Extraordinary Prognoses) make a reappearance here as required reading. We never do hear about the Four Virtues.

---

* Originally a term that meant the grain or texture of jade that must be followed while sculpting (SWJZ), (lǐ) 理 has come to mean "logic" or "reason." Not to be confused with (lǐ) 裡 "interior" which has a (yī) 衤 garment radical versus a (yù) 干 jade radical.

Discussion on Four Losses

徵四失論

(zhēng sì shī lùn)

In Chapter 78, Discussion on Four Losses, the Emperor tells Lei Gong of four more mistakes of practitioners. The Five Mistakes of the previous chapter are implied to be the fault of the practitioner, while these Four Losses sound more like limitations in talent or education. There are 12 jīng-channels and 365 luò-collaterals.

精神不專,
(jīng shén bù zhuān,)
[If the practitioner's] essence and spirit are not focused,

志意不理,
(zhì yì bù lǐ,)
willpower and intention are not orderly,

外內相失,
(wài nèi xiāng shī,)
outside and inside are mutually lost,

故時疑殆。

(gù shí yí dài.)

therefore sometimes [there will be] doubt and peril.

Four Losses

- Loss 1: Not knowing the counterflow and following of yin and yang

- Loss 2: Not completing one's studies, using too many modalities, believing in nonsense as if it were the Way, caring too much about reputation, haphazardly using biǎn stones

- Loss 3: Not adjusting to class and wealth, the thickness of the seat [cushion], the temperature of the body, the appropriateness of diet, not differentiating courage and timidity, and getting in one's own way. Not even knowing enough to know [one's inadequacies]

- Loss 4: Not asking the onset of disease, the disruption of emotions or diet, excesses of lifestyle, or possible poisoning, but diagnosing solely based on the radial pulse

The rest of the chapter is a few sentences of the Emperor lamenting how not knowing the Way to diagnose and treat properly brings gloom to brightness. The Emperor seems to lament a lot in these last chapters. Perhaps Qi Bo has passed away, or maybe the implementation of medicine through Lei Gong to benefit his subjects is less fun than studying the medicine with Qi Bo.

Discussion on Yin Yang Categories

陰陽類論

(yīn yáng lèi lùn)

Chapter 79, Discussion on Yin Yang Categories, is a conversation between the Emperor and Lei Gong on yin and yang.

Lei Gong thinks Liver is the most precious of the Five Zang

In the beginning of spring, the Emperor sits, looking upon the eight extremes, and the qi of (bā fēng) 八風 "eight winds,"* and asks Lei Gong, "Of the categories yin and yang, the Way of channels and vessels, the governance of five within [the body], which Zang is most precious?"

---

*   **Acu Trivia!** 八風 (bā fēng) "Eight Winds" is the name of the eight extra acupoints in the webbing of the toes.

Lei Gong answers, "Spring, of the first two heavenly stems, which governs Liver within, treated 72 days, is the season of vessels. Your vassal believes this Zang is most precious."

Six pulse signs

The Emperor responds cryptically with six pulses.

3 yang	Longitude 經 (jīng)	Taiyang	Radial pulse wiry, floating and does not sink
2 yang	Maintenance 維 (wéi)[190]	Yangming	Radial pulse wiry, deep, and not drum
1 yang	Wandering Area 游部 (yóu bù)	Shaoyang	Carotid pulse wiry, urgent, suspended
3 yin	Exterior 表 (biǎo)	Taiyin	Hidden drum not floating
2 yin	Interior 裡 (lǐ)	Arrives at Lung, qi belongs to Bladder, connects outside to Spleen and Stomach	
1 yin	New Moon Gloom 朔晦 (shuò huì)	Channel terminates, qi floats but not drum, hooked and slippery	

Following countenance, yin yang, and gender

Lei Gong seems to understand why his teacher answers this way, for he asks about (cóng róng) 從容 "following countenance," (yīn yáng) 陰陽 "yin yang," and (cí xióng) 雌雄 "gender."

The Emperor answers:

3 yang	Father 父 (fù)
2 yang	Defense 衛 (wèi)
1 yang	Record 紀 (jì)
3 yin	Mother 母 (mǔ)
2 yin	Female 雌 (cí)
1 yin	Lone Envoy 獨使 (dú shǐ)

Pulses mentioned in Chapter 79

2 yang + 1 yin	Yangming disease, all nine orifices sink
3 yang + 1 yin	Taiyang pulse excess, five Zang chaotic inside, (jīng hài) 驚駭 *Shock Terrors* outside
2 yin + 2 yang	Disease at Lung, Shaoyin pulse deep, Spleen and four limbs are harmed
2 yin + 2 yang	Disease at Kidney, (mà lì) 罵詈 *Cursing*, (wàng xíng) 妄行 *Frenetic Movement*, (diān jí) 巔疾 *Vertex Disease*, and (kuáng) 狂 *Mania*
2 yin + 1 yang	Disease from Kidney, yin qi lingers in Heart, digestive organs descend empty orifices, embankment (bì sè bù tōng) 閉塞不通 *No Throughput*, four limbs separate
1 yin + 1 yang	Yin qi arrives at Heart, disregulation above and below, unaware of ingestion and elimination, throat dry, disease at Earth/Spleen
2 yang + 3 yin	Yin cannot surpass yang, yang cannot stop yin, float becomes (xiě jiǎ) 血瘕 *Blood Conglomeration*, sink becomes (nóng fǔ) 膿胕 *Pus Rot*

Death prognoses

Lei Gong asks about something called (duǎn qī) 短期 "short dates" which I believe has to do with death prognoses.* The Emperor does not answer. Lei Gong asks again. The Emperor says, "It is in the classical discussions."†

Lei Gong, ever patient, rephrases his question, "Please may I hear about short dates?"

The Emperor states, "Disease of the three winter months, when combined with yang, will exhibit death signs in the first month of spring. Disease of the three winter months, when reason is exhausted, grass and willow leaves have died, yin and yang both terminate in spring, [death] date in early spring. Disease of the three spring months, known as (yáng shā) 陽殺 *Yang Killing*, yin and yang both terminate, [death] date when grass dries. Disease of the three summer months, not more

---

*   短期 (duǎn qī) "short date"...in Chinese culture, (duǎn) 短 "short" is
    sometimes used as a euphemism for death.

†   What a jerk! I despise power dynamics that play out this way.

than ten days past Ultimate Yin, (yīn yáng jiāo) 陰陽交 *Yin-Yang Exchange*, [death] date when water freezes. Disease of the three autumn months, three yang arise simultaneously, and recovery may occur without treatment. Those with *Yin-Yang Exchange* cannot sit down from standing, cannot stand up after sitting. If three yang arrive alone, [death] date at (shí shuǐ) 石水 'Stone Water.' If two yin arrive alone, date at (shèng shuǐ) 盛水 'Abundant Water.'" I thought *Stone Water* was a disease name, but in this line both Stone Water and Abundant Water seem like a marking of time.

Discussion on Measuring Abundance and Decline

方盛衰論

(fāng shèng shuāi lùn)

Chapter 80 is entitled Discussion on Measuring Abundance and Decline.

Quantity of qi, counterflow, and following

Lei Gong asks about the quantity of qi, and which indicates (nì) 逆 "counterflow," which indicates (cóng) 從 "following."

The Emperor answers, "Yang follows left, yin follows right. Age follows up, youth follows down. Therefore spring and summer belong to yang and life. [That which] belongs to autumn and winter dies. Reverse this, and that which belongs to autumn and winter lives, therefore any amount of counterflow qi counts as (jué) 厥 *Reversal*."

[Lei Gong] asks, "So (yǒu yú) 有餘 *Excess* is (jué) 厥 *Reversal*?"

[The Emperor] answers, "[If] one ascends and does not descend, the (hán jué) 寒厥 *Cold Reversal* reaches the knees. A young patient will die in autumn and winter, an aged patient will live through autumn and winter. If qi ascends but does not descend, (tóu tòng) 頭痛 *Headache* and (diān jí) 巔疾 *Vertex Disease* [will occur]. Yang cannot be gotten, yin cannot be discerned...therefore (shǎo qì zhī jué) 少氣之厥 *Reversal of Scant Qi* makes a person have crazy dreams until she or he is ultimately confused. [When the] three yang terminate, three yin faint, this is known as (shǎo qì) 少氣 *Scant Qi*.

Dream interpretations: deficiency

~ Qi deficiency	Dream imagery ([occurs] in corresponding season)
Lung	White objects, bloody beheadings (armies battling)
Kidney	Shipwreck, drownings (hiding fearfully submerged in water)
Liver	Fragrant mushrooms and herbs (lying under a tree not daring to get up)
Heart	Fire rescue, yang objects (uncontrolled burning)
Spleen	Not enough food and water (constructing walls and buildings)

All these dreamscapes are caused by qi deficiency in the five Zang, excess yang qi, insufficient yin qi. Regulate the yin and yang through the jīng-channels and mài-vessels.

Ten degrees of diagnosis

There are 10 (duó) 度 "degrees" of diagnosis: pulse, Zang, flesh, sinew, cave/acupoint measure. They are not explained here. Instead, there is a long passage about misdiagnosis and potential consequences, followed by an explanation of what sages must know in diagnosis, including but not limited to: the ugly and the kind, diseased and unafflicted, high and low, seated and risen, start and stop.

Death signs and diagnosis admonishments

If the body is weak and qi is deficient, death [occurs]. If the form has excess qi and the vessels' qi (pulse?) is insufficient, death. If there is excess in the vessels but insufficiency in the form, live. Therefore, there are general guidelines to diagnosis, regularity to sitting and rising (i.e. lifestyle), movement to coming and going in order to turn the (shén míng) 神明 "spirit clarity," [one] must be clear and clean, observe above and below, discern the eight uprights and evils, differentiate the five areas in the middle, press the pulse for motion and stillness, follow the chǐ for slippery and choppy, cold and warmth, view the size [of the pulse] and combine it with symptoms of counterflow and following to know the name of the disease, and have a perfect diagnosis that does not miss human emotion. Therefore, diagnosis involves viewing the breath, the intention, not missing the moment to treat, the way is to be bright in observation in order to last long. If one does not know this way, one loses the channel and terminates reason, speak of perishing on absurd dates; this is known as 失道 (shī dào) "Losing the Way."

Discussion Explaining Essential Subtleties

解精微論

(jiě jīng wēi lùn)

Chapter 81, Discussion Explaining Essential Subtleties, though supposedly another lesson for Lei Gong, seems to be really about the mystery of tears and the anatomy of weeping.

Lei Gong asks about those who weep but do not shed tears versus those who weep few tears and have scanty snot.

The Emperor answers snottily, (zài jīng yǒu yě) 「在經有也。」 "It is in the classics." A pun for "in the channels," since both (jīng diǎn) 經典 "classics" and (jīng mài) 經脈 "meridian vessels" use the same character (jīng) 經.

The anatomy of tears

Lei Gong inquires again, "[I] do not know where the water comes from."

The Emperor, after disparaging this question as not applicable to treatment, explains the anatomy of tears. "Heart is the focus of the five Zangs' jīng-essence; the eye is its orifice; the complexion is its glory. Therefore, if a person is virtuous, then qi is harmonious within the eyes; if misfortune happens, worry can be known via the complexion. Therefore when there is sadness tears descend. The accumulation of water is (zhì yīn) 至陰 'Ultimate Yin';* Ultimate Yin is the jīng-essence of Kidney. Under normal circumstances, the ancestral jīng water does not exude because the jīng-essence holds it, supporting and wrapping it to keep it from flowing. The jīng-essence of water is zhì-willpower. The essence of fire is shén-spirit. When water and fire affect each other to make both shén and zhì sad, (mù zhī shuǐ) 目之水 'waters of the eyes' (i.e. tears) are generated. Thus the proverb: 'Heart sadness is called (zhì bēi) 志悲 *Emotional Grief.* Willpower[†] and heart essence both gather at the eyes.' Therefore, grief passes its qi to the heart. Essence ascends and does not pass to the will. And will grieves alone, producing tears."

The relationship between tears and snot

"(Qì) 泣 'tears' and (tì) 涕 'snot' are brains. Brains are yin, marrow, that which fills the bones. Therefore (nǎo shèn) 腦滲 *Brain Seepage* becomes snot. Will is governed by bone, therefore tears followed by snot are of a kind. Snot and tears are like human brothers; they live and die together. This is why tears and snot flow out together when a woman cries, because they are of a kind."

Weeping without tears explained

Lei Gong repeats his original question about weeping without tears, or without much snot following.

---

*   **Acu Trivia!** (zhì yīn) 至陰 "Ultimate Yin" is the name of UB67.

†   志 (zhì): "willpower" as related to Kidney, and "emotion/feeling" in general.

The Emperor responds, "If there are no tears, the weeping is (bù bēi) 不悲 'not grief,' i.e. not due to grief or sadness. If there is no weeping, the shén-spirit has no compassion. When the spirit is not compassionate, the will is not sad. If yin and yang hold each other, where do tears come from? One who has *Willpower Grief* regrets. Regret rushes yin. Rushing yin makes willpower exit through the eyes. [When] willpower leaves the eyes, then shén-spirit cannot guard jīng-essence, jīng [and] shén go to the eyes, and tears and snot are exuded. (jué) 厥 *Reversal* causes (mù wú suǒ jiàn) 目無所見 *Blindness*. When a person has (jué) 厥 *Reversal*, her yang qi will bìng-merge above, yin qi will bìng-merge below. When yang bìng-merge above then candleflame lights;* when yin bìng-merge below then the feet are cold. Cold feet causes (zhàng) 胀 *Distension*."

Tearing up in the wind

"Therefore one water cannot best five fires, and the canthus is blinded. This is why the eyes tear up endlessly in the wind, because eyes in wind guard yang qi within the jīng-essence. It is fire qi that burns the eyes which causes them to tear up in the wind. Similarly, fire generates wind, making rain possible."

---

* 「火燭光也」 (huǒ zhú guāng yě) "fire candle light end-of-sentence-flag." Does this mean the patient is sensitive to light?

Acknowledgments

My deepest thanks to Cassandra Segal for test reading and commentary, to Jiǎng Lè 蔣樂 and Zhāng Shànjūn 張善君 Adela Chang for bilingual proofreading and commentary, to Dr. Henry McCann for mentoring me on the doctoral capstone project that became the first draft of this book, to Rachel and Gideon Guaraldi for sharing their log cabin in Vermont as a doctoral writing retreat center in August of 2017, to Melissa Illingworth and Jessica Frier for proofreading the original capstone, to Claire Wilson and the staff at Singing Dragon Press, to Robi Robinson for last minute formatting, to Sydney Malawer for proofreading, to Lisa Ozaeta for helping me figure out how to type pinyin tones on my laptop, to Judith Lyn Sutton for instilling in me a love of writing and the skills needed to revise and proofread a manuscript for publication, and to Kate Sassoon, who lived with my piles of reference materials, did all my chores and reminded me to eat through the seemingly endless months of reading, writing and re-writing.

Profound gratitude also to all my classmates at the Oregon College of Oriental Medicine who inspired and encouraged me in the beginning, and to my students at the Acupuncture and Integrative Medicine College in Berkeley who have seen me through to the end.

Last but not least, I am most gratefully indebted to my mother's mother, Yè Kěhuá 葉可華, for instilling native Chinese fluency in her eldest granddaughter, without which this book could not have been possible.

Appendices

Appendix A: Diagram of the Generating and Controlling Cycles

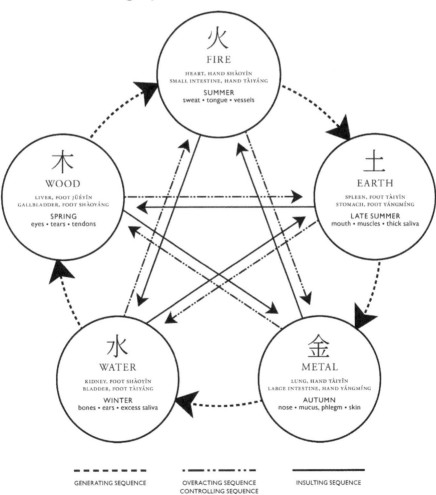

火
FIRE

HEART, HAND SHÀOYĪN
SMALL INTESTINE, HAND TÀIYÁNG

SUMMER
sweat • tongue • vessels

木
WOOD

LIVER, FOOT JÜÉYĪN
GALLBLADDER, FOOT SHÀOYÁNG

SPRING
eyes • tears • tendons

土
EARTH

SPLEEN, FOOT TÀIYĪN
STOMACH, FOOT YÁNGMÍNG

LATE SUMMER
mouth • muscles • thick saliva

水
WATER

KIDNEY, FOOT SHÀOYĪN
BLADDER, FOOT TÀIYÁNG

WINTER
bones • ears • excess saliva

金
METAL

LUNG, HAND TÀIYĪN
LARGE INTESTINE, HAND YÁNGMÍNG

AUTUMN
nose • mucus, phlegm • skin

GENERATING SEQUENCE

OVERACTING SEQUENCE
CONTROLLING SEQUENCE

INSULTING SEQUENCE

Appendix B. Glossary of Chinese Terms (in alphabetical order by pinyin, homonyms in order of tone and appearance in the text)

Key:
《Chinese》 <u>Book Name</u>
(*category*)
[clarifications]
disease, sign/symptom
<notes from the author/other annotators>
Proper Names (date of birth-date of death)
(Other expert: definition(s) which differ
    from Amy's)
「Chinese quote」 'Complete sentence
    translation.'
"transliteration"
/ = and/or
? = could not find satisfactory definition
i.e. = in other words

ài 愛 love, beloved
ān 安 to calm
ān jìng 安靜 peace [and] quiet (*governance of earth*)
ān níng 安寧 calm, tranquil
àn qiào 按蹻 pressing the [Yin/Yang] Qiao, i.e. bodywork

bā 八 eight
bā fēng 八風 Eight Winds, acupoints M-LE-8
bā liáo 八髎 Eight Foramen, acupoints Bladder 31-34
bā xié 八邪 Eight Evils, acupoints M-UE-22
bǎi 百 hundred
Bái Shì Nèijīng 《白氏內經》 <u>White Clan's Internal Classic</u>
Bái Shì Pángpiān 《白氏旁篇》 <u>White Clan's Side Articles</u>
Bái Shì Wàijīng 《白氏外經》 <u>White Clan's External Classic</u>

bái zhú 白朮 white atractylodes rhizome, atractylodis macrocephalae rhizoma
bāo bì 胞痹 *uterus impediment*
bāo luò 胞絡 uterus collateral (Wiseman: uterine network vessels)
bāo luò jué 胞絡絕 *uterus collateral vanishing*
bāo mài 胞脈 uterus vessel
bàn 半 half
Bān Gù 班固 (32-92) historian, politician, and poet, author of the <u>Book of Han</u>
Bān Zhāo 班昭 (45-116) Ban Gu's younger sister who finished writing the <u>Book of Han</u> after his death
bǎo 寶 treasure
bào bìng 暴病 violent illness, i.e. acute disease
bào jīng 暴驚 *violent shock*
bào jué 暴厥 *violent reversal* (Wiseman: fulminant reversal)
bào lóng 暴聾 *violent deafness*
bào luán 暴攣 *violent contraction*
bào luán wěi bì 暴攣痿痹 *violent contraction/atrophy/impediment*
bào nù 暴怒 *violent anger*
bào sǐ 暴死 *violent death*, i.e. sudden death
bào tòng 暴痛 *violent pain*, i.e. acute pain
bào xǐ 暴喜 *violent joy*
bào yīn 暴瘖 *violent aphonia*
bào zhàng 暴脹 *violent distension*
bào zhù 暴注 *violent diarrhea*
bēi 悲 sadness
bèi 背 [upper] back
běi 北 north
bèi 備 to prepare, also one zhōu-circuit of sky's qì-node, i.e. six ji-years
běi fēng 北風 north wind
bèi huà 備化 prepared transformation (*even earth year name*)

bēi jiān 卑監 inferior supervisor (insufficient earth year name)

bèi lǚ jīn tòng 背脊筋痛 back sinew pain

bèi nèi 背內 Inner Spine, alternate acupoint name for Bladder 11

bèi shū 背俞 [Upper] Back Shu, alternate acupoint name for Bladder 12

bèi tòng 背痛 [upper] back pain

bēi wàng 悲妄 sadness/grief-induced delirium

běn 本 root

běn bìng 本病 root disease

běn shū 本輸 original transporter acupoints, i.e. jǐng-well, yíng-spring, shū-stream, jīng- river, hé-sea

Běnbìng 《本病》 Root Diseases

Běnjīng 《本經》 Roots Classic, nickname of the Shennong Bencao Jing

bēng 崩 avalanche [menorrhagia] (Wiseman: flooding)

bí 鼻 nose

bǐ 彼 other, that

bì 閉 shut (Wiseman: block)

bì 痹 impediment

bì 必 must, require

bì 臂 arm

bì 髀 femur

bì 壁 eastwall (Chinese constellation)

bì 畢 fork (Chinese constellation)

bì bì 痹躄 impediment lameness

bì bù tōng 閉不通 [urinary] block and inhibition

bì cáng 閉藏 shut and hide, or closed and hidden

bì qì 痹氣 impediment qi

bí qiú 鼻鼽 nasal congestion (Wiseman: sniveling)

bì sāi 閉塞 blockage and congestion (Wiseman: block)

bì sè bù tōng 閉塞不通 no throughput

bì wài lián tòng 臂外廉痛 lateral arm pain

bí yuān 鼻淵 nasal discharge

biāo 標 branch, literally "treetop" (Wiseman: tip)

biāo běn 標本 root and branch (Wiseman: root and tip)

biǎo 表 exterior

biǎo lǐ 表裡 exterior-interior

biàn 變 change (Wiseman: transmutation)

biàn huà 變化 change and transformation (Wiseman: mutation)

biǎn shí 砭石 bloodletting stones

Biǎn Què Nèijīng 《扁鵲內經》 Bian Que's Internal Classic

Biǎn Què Wàijīng 《扁鵲外經》 Bian Que's External Classic

bié 別 divergent, separated

bié lùn 別論 addendum

bǐng 稟 endowed [by]

bǐng 丙 3rd heavenly stem

bìng 病 disease

bìng 并 parallel

bìng chuán 病傳 pathophysiology (Wiseman: disease shift)

bìng fēng 病風 disease [of] wind

bìng jī 病機 pathogenesis (Wiseman: pathomechanism)

bìng jī shí jiǔ tiáo 病機十九條 19 Lines of Pathogenesis (Wiseman: Nineteen Pathomechanisms)

bìng wēn 病溫 disease [that is] warm

bìng zhě 病者 patient, literally "diseased one"

bìng zhī cháng 病之常 commonalities of disease

bìng zhōng 病中 disease [in] middle

bó 搏 contend, struck [in combat], brawl

bǒ 跛 limp

bó jué 薄厥 thin reversal (Wiseman: vehement reversal)

bǔ 補 to mend, patch, supplement, tonify

bù 不 not, no, none [pronounced bú when appearing before another 4th tone]

bù 布 (v.) to spread [like a sheet of fabric]

bù 部 (v.) to separate into sections, area

bù ān 不安 unrest, unrestful, unpeaceful

bú bì qīn shū 不避親疎 does not respect boundaries

bù dé 不得 cannot [get], limited

bù hé 不和 not harmonious, no harmony

bù jí 不及 not up to, not reaching, i.e. insufficient

bù kě (yǐ) 不可(以) not allowed, i.e. don't, can't

bú lè 不樂 lacking joy

bú lì 不利 inhibited, inhibition

bù néng 不能 cannot

bú rèn 不任 not voluntary, unable to, i.e. dysfunctional

bù rén 不仁 numbness, from nutritive qi deficiency, literally "not benevolent" or "no sensation"

bú shì shí 不嗜食 low appetite, literally "no addiction [to] food"

bù shí wò 不時臥 sleep at odd hours, irregular sleep, literally "no time [to] lie supine"

bù shōu 不收 inability to contract

bú tuì wèi 不退位 (chronobiology term related to running early)

bù xiū 不休 unceasingly

bù xǔ 不許 not allowed, i.e. nonconsensual

bú yòng 不用 no function, from defensive qi deficiency

bú yù shí 不欲食 *not desiring food*, i.e. low appetite

bú yuè 不月 no moon/monthly, i.e. amenorrhea

bú yùn 不孕 no pregnancy, i.e. *infertility*

bù zhī 不知 not knowing

bú zhì 不治 not treatable

bù zú 不足 insufficiency, literally "not enough"

cāng 蒼 blue-gray

cáng 藏 hide or hidden [as in treasure]

cāng lǐn 倉廩 granary

cāng yǔn 蒼隕 age [and] perish [as in a falling meteor] *(catastrophe of metal)*

cāng zhú 蒼朮 blue-gray atractylodes rhizome, atractylodis rhizoma

cè 測 measure

chán zhēn 鑱鍼 the 1st of 9 needles listed in Chapter 1 of the <u>Lingshu</u>

chāng 昌 prosper

cháng 腸 intestine, intestines

cháng 常 common, normal, regular

cháng 长 long, extended

cháng bì 腸痹 *intestinal impediment*

cháng fēng 腸風 *intestinal wind*

cháng jiǔ 長久 sustainability

cháng míng 腸鳴 *borborygmus*

cháng qì 常氣 regular qi

cháng pì 腸澼 *intestinal blockage* (Wiseman: intestinal aggregation)

chāng yáng 昌陽 Prosperous Yang, alternate acupoint name for Kidney 7 (Wiseman: Glorious Yang)

chēn 䐜 *bloating*

chēn 瘨 abscess <Amy and Huángfǔ Mì: probably a copying error.>

chén 陳 aged

chén 沈 sinking

chén 臣 deputy [herb] (Wiseman: minister)

chén 辰 5th earthly branch, 7-9am, 4/5-5/4, year of the Dragon, compass point 120°

chén pí 陳皮 aged tangerine skin

chén shǐ 臣使 jester

chēn zhàng 䐜脹 *bloating distension*

chǐ 尺 unit of measurement equal to 10 cùn, also a proximal radial pulse position, i.e. cubit

chǐ 齒 tooth, teeth

chǐ chún hán tòng 齒唇寒痛 *teeth/lips cold pain*

chǐ qǔ 齒齲 *tooth decay*

chōng 沖 rush

chōng mài 沖脈 the Penetrating Vessel (Wiseman: thoroughfare vessel)

chōng shàn 沖疝 *rushing hernia*

chōng yáng 衝陽 Rushing Yang, acupoint Stomach 42

chén 陳 aged

chéng 成 become, complete, accomplish

chéng qì tāng 承氣湯 formula family from the <u>Shanghan Lun</u>, containing dà huáng for laxative effect

chì 瘈 *clonic convulsion*

chì 赤 scarlet red

chóng 重 double

chóng fāng 重方 double formula

chóng fù zhǒng 重跗腫 *bilateral foot edema*

chóng shí 重實 double excess, occurs when erroneously tonified during full moon

chóng yáng 重陽 double yang

chóng yīn 重陰 double yin

chǒu 丑 2nd earthly branch, 1-3am, 1/6-2/3, year of the Ox, compass point 30°

chū 出 to exit

chū 初 beginning

chù 處 location

chuǎn 喘 *panting* (Wiseman: dyspnea)

chuǎn 腨 calf

chuán dào 傳道 passkeeper, literally "[one who] spreads/passes on the Way"

chuǎn hū 喘呼 *asthma*, literally "panting exhalations"

chuǎn ké 喘欬 *panting cough* (Wiseman: pant and cough)

chuán huà zhī fǔ 傳化之府 the transformational Fu-organs

chuán xī 喘息 *panting audibly*

chuāng 瘡 *sore*

chuāng 窗 window in a dwelling

chuāng yáng 瘡瘍 *ulcers/sores*

chūn 春 spring *(season)*

chún 唇 lips

chún 淳 pure, honest

chūn fēn 春分 spring equinox *(solar term)*

cí 雌 female

cǐ 此 this

cì 刺 (v.) to prick, poke, needle; (n.) acupuncture

cì fǎ 刺法 pricking methods, i.e. acupuncture techniques/prescriptions

cì jiā 刺家 acupuncturist, literally "specialist/person who pricks"

cí xióng 雌雄 gender, sex, literally "female male"

cǐ zhī wèi yě 「此之謂也」 'This is what we're talking about.'

cóng 從 (v.) to follow, go with the flow, (p.) from

cóng gé 從革 *(insufficient metal year name)*
cóng róng 從容 following countenance
còu lǐ 腠理 interstices
cù 卒 sudden
cù xīn tòng 卒心痛 *sudden angina*
cù shàn 卒疝 *sudden hernia* (Wiseman: sudden mounting)
cù tòng 卒痛 *sudden pain*
cuàn 篡 usurp (Wiseman: perineum)
cuì 脆 brittle, crunchy, crisp
cún 存 to store or preserve
cùn 寸 unit of measurement equal to one thumb-width, also distal radial pulse position, i.e. inch
cūn jiē 皴揭 *chapped skin*
cùn kǒu 寸口 radial pulse
cuó 痤 *acne*
cuó fèi 痤痱 *acne rash* (Wiseman: pock pimples)

dá 達 to arrive, achieve, attain, reach
dà 大 great, or big
dà bì 大痹 *large impediment*
dà dīng 大疔 *big boil*
dà fēng 大風 *big wind*
dà jiǎ 大瘕 *big conglomeration*
dà jī 大積 *great accumulations*
dà jù 大聚 *great gatherings*
dà lùn 大論 big discussion, i.e. treatise
dà lóu 大傻 *hunchback*
dà luò 大絡 great connector, designation of Spleen 21 *dàbāo* and apical pulse *xūlǐ*
dà qì 大氣 big qi, i.e. atmosphere
dà zé 大則 general/great principle
dà zhuī 大椎 Big Vertebrae, acupoint Du 14, also the name of the C7 vertebrae
Dà Yào 《大要》 Big Essentials
dà yíng 大迎 Great Welcome, acupoint Stomach 5, also the hollow of the jawbone
dà zhù 大杼 Big Loom-shuttle, acupoint Bladder 11 (Wiseman: Great Shuttle)
dà bāo 大包 Big Hug, acupoint Spleen 21 (Wiseman: Great Embracement)
dà dūn 大敦 Big and Grounded, Liver 1 (Wiseman: Large Pile)
dài 殆 peril
dài 待 to await
dài 帶 belt, short for Belt Vessel, 4th of the 8 Extraordinary Vessels
dài mài 帶脈 Belt Vessel (Wiseman: girdling vessel)
dài xià 帶下 leukorrhea, vaginal discharge, literally "belt descending"
dān 癉 *drought* (Wiseman: pure heat)
dān 丹 cinnabar

dān nuè 癉瘧 *drought ague* (Wiseman: pure-heat malaria)
dàn zhōng 膻中 Sternum Center, acupoint Ren 17 (Wiseman: chest center)
dāng 當 should
dǎo 導 to direct, guide
dǎo 倒 to invert or reverse
dào 道 pathway, the Way
dǎo yǐn 導引 guided exercise
dǎn 膽 gallbladder
dàn 旦 dawn
dǎn dān 膽癉 *gallbladder drought*
dǎn mù 膽募 "gallbladder front-mu", i.e. acupoint Gallbladder 24
dǎn shū 膽俞 "gallbladder back-shu", i.e. acupoint Bladder 19
dé 德 virtue
dé 得 to get, acquire
dé hòu yǔ qì 得後與氣 *passing stools and gas*
dé qì 得氣 getting qi, i.e. needling to disperse
dī 氐 dragonfoot *(Chinese constellation)*
dì 地 land, ground, country, geography
dì 帝 emperor, short for Huángdì
dì cāng 地蒼 a greenish black color, also Land Blue-Gray, acupoint Stomach 4
dì lǐ 地理 geography
dì qì 地氣 land qi, i.e. geographic qi
dì sè 地色 the color of ground
dì zhī 地支 [12] earthly branches
diǎn 點 point, a dot on a line
diān bìng 癲病 *withdrawal disease*, i.e. epilepsy
diān jí 癲疾 *vertex disease* (Wiseman: disease of the head)
diān kuáng 癲狂 *withdrawal/mania* (Wiseman: mania and withdrawal)
dīng 丁 4th heavenly stem
dǐng 頂 crown of head
dìng 定 fix(ed), stabilize, set
dōng 冬 winter *(season)*
dōng 東 east
dòng 動 move
dōng hàn 東漢 Eastern Han [Dynasty] (25-220)
dōng fēng 東風 east wind
dòng xiè 洞泄 *grotto diarrhea* (Wiseman: thoroughflux diarrhea)
dòu ér zhù zhuī 「鬥而鑄錐」 forge weapons during battle *(proverb)*
dū 都 capital or big city
dú 瀆 ditch, sluice
dú 毒 poison, toxin
dú 獨 alone, solitary

dù 度 measurement, also a unit of measurement equal to two vertebral heights

dú bí 犢鼻 Baby Ox Nose, acupoint Stomach 35 (Wiseman: Calfs Nose)

dù liáng 度量 degrees [and] measurements

dū mài 督脈 Governing Vessel

dú shǐ 獨使 lone envoy

dú yào 毒藥 toxic herbs

dú zhì 獨至 arrives alone

duān 端 standing upright

duǎn 短 short *(pulse texture)*, also sometimes used as a euphemism for death/dying

duàn 斷 to judge, break

duǎn qī 短期 short dates, short duration

duì yuē 對曰 (v.) answers, replies

dūn 敦 groundedness, honest, trustworthy

dūn fù 敦阜 grounded/honest mound *(excess earth year name)*

duō 多 many, more, profuse

duó 度 degree(s)

duō hàn 多汗 *profuse sweat*

duó xiě 奪血 *stolen blood*

ér 而 and then

ěr 耳 ear

èr 二 two

ěr lóng 耳聾 *deafness*

ěr míng 耳鳴 *tinnitus*

èr shí yī 二十一 21

ěr wú suǒ wén 耳無所聞 *inability to hear*

èr yīn 二陰 two yin [orifices], i.e. urethral opening and anus

ěr zhōng shēng fēng 耳中生風 *wind inside the ear*, i.e. tinnitus

fā 發 express or release

fá 伐 to chop

fǎ 髮 hair

fǎ 法 law, method

fā chén 發陳 release the aged

fā jī 發機 release mechanism

fā rè 發熱 *express heat*, can mean fever or subjective sensations

fā shēng 發生 express birth *(excess wood year name)*

fán 蕃 flourish

fán 煩 vexation

fán 凡 all, whatever

fǎn 反 reverse, opposite, flip side

fàn 犯 offend, attack, invade

fǎn cè 反側 extension/lateral rotation

fán mǎn 煩滿 *vexation fullness* (Wiseman: vexation and fullness)

fán mào 蕃茂 flourish luxuriance *(transformation of fire)*

fán ruò 燔焫 blaze [and] ignite *(catastrophe of fire)*

fán xiù 蕃秀 flourish and fecundate

fán yuān 煩冤 *vexation grievance* (Wiseman: vexation and low spirits)

fǎn zhé 反折 *tonic spasm* [of the Du Mai]

fǎn zuǒ 反佐 reverse envoy

fāng 方 square, direction, approach, [herbal] formula

fāng yí 方宜 appropriate methods

fēi 非 not

féi 肥 fat, flabby

fèi 肺 lung

fèi 痱 rash

fèi bì 肺痹 *lung impediment*

fèi fēng 肺風 *lung wind*

fèi fēng shàn 肺風疝 *lung wind hernia*

féi guì rén 肥貴人 fat highborn person

fèi shàn 肺疝 *lung hernia* (Wiseman: lung mounting)

fèi xiāo 肺消 *lung wasting* (Wiseman: lung dispersion)

fèi yáng 飛揚 Fly and Soar, acupoint Bladder 58

fēn 分 separate, divide, also a unit of measurement approximately 0.375 grams or 0.1 cùn

fēn bù 分部 designated areas

fēn lǐ 分理 muscle interstices

fēn ròu 分肉 Divide Flesh, alternate acupoint name for Gallbladder 36

fēng 風 wind

fēng 封 seal

fēng chí 風池 Wind Pond, acupoint Gallbladder 20 (Wiseman: Wind Pool)

fēng fǔ 風府 Wind Mansion, acupoint Du 16

fēng jué 風厥 *wind reversal*

fēng nuè 風瘧 *wind ague* (Wiseman: wind malaria)

fēng rè 風熱 *wind-heat*

fēng shuǐ 風水 *wind water*

fēng xiāo 風消 *wind wasting* (Wiseman: wind dispersion)

fǒu 否 refute, reject

fū 膚 surface

fū 夫 classic flagword at the beginning of sentence to introduce new topic

fū 跗 dorsum of foot

fú 浮 floating

fú 伏 hidden [in ambush], conceal, lie low

fú 福 prosperity, good fortune, blessing

fǔ 府 Yang Organ (Unschuld: palace, Wiseman: Bowel)

fǔ 甫 honorific term for a great man, literally "sprouting field"

fǔ 俛 flexion

fù 父 father

fù 腹 abdomen

fù 復 retaliation, revenge, recovery, reply

fú bái 浮白 Floating White, acupoint Gallbladder 10

fù bù 復布 *(chronobiology term related to running late)*

fù dà 腹大 *abdomen enlarged*

fū hé 敷和 applied harmony *(virtue of wood)*

fū hé 敷合 applied convergence *(even wood year name)*

fú liáng 伏梁 *hidden roofbeam* (Wiseman: deep-lying beam)

fù mǎn 腹滿 *abdominal fullness*

fú míng 伏明 hidden brightness *(insufficient fire year name)*

fù mǔ 父母 parents

fù rén 婦人 woman

fù tòng 腹痛 *abdominal pain*

fú tú 扶突 Support Protrusion, acupoint Large Intestine 18 (Wiseman: protuberance assistant)

fú tù 伏兔 Hidden Bunny, acupoint Stomach 31 (Wiseman: crouching rabbit)

fú xū 浮虛 *floating emptiness* (Wiseman: vacuous puffiness, also qi swelling)

fǔ yǎng 俛仰 flex and extend

fú yún 浮雲 floating clouds

fù zhàng 腹脹 *abdominal distension*

fù zhī mǎn 腹支滿 *abdominal propping fullness*

fù zhǒng 跗腫 *dorsum [of foot] swelling*

fú zhǒng 浮腫 *superficial swelling*

fǔ zhǒng 腐腫 *rot swelling*

fù zhǒng 腹腫 *abdominal swelling*

fù zhǒng 跗腫 *puffy swelling*, i.e. edema

fū zǐ 夫子 honorific term of address for a teacher [as in Kǒng-fūzǐ 孔夫子 Confucius]

fù zǐ 附子 aconite root

gài 蓋 to cover

gān 肝 liver

gān 乾 dry

gān 干 interfere, offend

gān 甘 sweet

gǎn 感 to be affected by

gān bì 肝痺 *liver impediment*

gān fēng 肝風 *liver wind*

gān fēng shàn 肝風疝 *liver wind hernia*

gān xū 肝虛 liver deficiency

gāng 綱 headrope of a fishing net, i.e. outline, principle

gāng 剛 rigid

gāo gǔ 高骨 high bone, i.e. radial styloid process or lumbar vertebrae

gé 隔 *block* [at the diaphragm], i.e. continuous vomiting

gé 膈 diaphragm

gé 格 *repel*, alternate character for 隔 when it means continuous vomiting

gè 各 each

gé huāng 隔肓 diaphragmatic membrane <Note from Amy: I believe the characters 隔 and 膈 are used interchangeably for diaphragm.>

gé yáng 格陽 repelled yang

gé zhōng 隔中 blocked middle [jiao]

gēn 根 root

gēn shí 根蝕 root corrosion

gēng 庚 7th heavenly stem

gōng 功 success, achievement

gōng 工 work, craftsman, practitioner

gōng 宮 1st note on musical scale, roughly equivalent to Do

gòng 共 collectively, altogether

Gōngsūn Xuānyuán 公孫軒轅 Huangdi's actual name

gōu 鉤 hook *(pulse texture)*

gǔ 骨 bone, bones

gǔ 蠱 *possession*

gǔ 股 buttock (Wiseman: thigh)

gù 故 therefore; (n.) past, former

gù 顧 to turn around and look, i.e. lateral rotation of the neck

gù 固 harden, solidify (Wiseman: secure)

gǔ bì 骨痺 *bone impediment*

gǔ bù shōu 股不收 *gluteals not contracting*

gǔ jié biàn 骨節變 *bony joint derangement*

gǔ suí 骨髓 bone and marrow

gǔ tòng 骨痛 *bone pain*

gǔ wěi 骨痿 *bone atrophy* (Wiseman: bone wilting)

gǔ zhàng 鼓脹 *drum distension*

gǔ zhòng 骨重 *bone heaviness*

guā lóu shí 瓜蔞實 trichosanthes fruit (herb)

guān 觀 observe

guān 官 official

guān 關 gate (of a city), mountain pass, the middle radial pulse position, i.e. bar; also short for joint 關節 (guān jié) and *urinary stoppage* disease

guàn hàn 灌汗 *pouring sweat*

guān gé 關格 *block and repulsion*

guān shū 關樞 gate hinge, yang of taiyang skin area

guān yīn 關陰 blocked yin

guān yuán 關元 Gate Origin, acupoint Ren 4 (Wiseman: pass head)

guān zhé 關蟄 gate of hibernating insects, yin of taiyin skin area

guāng 光 light, luster, can also mean naked

guǎng míng 廣明 broad brighness

guī 歸 to return

guǐ 鬼 ghost (Chinese constellation)

guǐ 癸 10th heavenly stem

guì 貴 valuable

guī shén 鬼神 superstitiousness

Guǐyú Qū 鬼臾區 the Yellow Emperor's chronobiology teacher

guó 國 kingdom

guó 膕 popliteal crease

guò 過 [to go] too far, i.e. excess; also (n.) mistake(s)

hǎi 海 sea, ocean

hài 亥 12th earthly stem, 9-11pm, 11/7-12/6, year of the Boar, compass point 330°

hài fēi 害蜚 "harmful cockroach" i.e. yang of yangming collateral varicosities

hái guān 骸關 knee joint

hài jiān 害肩 harm shoulder, yin of pericardium skin area

hǎi zǎo 海藻 sargassum seaweed

hào 耗 spent, consumed (Wiseman: wear)

hào 好 (v.) prefers to

hán 寒 cold

hàn 汗 sweat

hán biàn 寒變 *cold changes*

hàn chū 汗出 sweating, literally "sweat exits"

hán fǔ 寒府 Cold Mansion, alternate acupoint name for Gallbladder 33

hán jí 寒疾 cold ailment

hán jué 寒厥 *cold reversal*

hán lì 寒慄 *cold shivers*

hán nuè 寒瘧 *cold ague* (Wiseman: cold malaria)

hán rè 寒熱 *cold [and] heat*

hán yáng 寒瘍 *cold sores*

hán zhì 寒至 cold arrival, i.e. pathogenic cold arrives during cold weather

hán zhòng 寒中 *cold stroke*

hán zhòng cháng míng 寒中腸鳴 **cold strike borborygmus**

Hàn Shū 《漢書》 Book of Han

hé 合 convergence [same character as hé-sea point]

hé 和 harmony, to harmonize

hé 闔 door-leaf

hé 核 core

hé fēi 闔飛 door-leaf flying, alternate characters for 害蜚 (hài fēi) yang of yangming collateral varicosities

hé liú 涸流 desiccated flow *(insufficient water year name)*

hé wèi 何謂 what is the meaning of

hè xī 赫曦 awe-inspiring early morning sunlight *(excess fire year name)*

hé yě 何也 why [is this]?

Hé Yùjī 《合玉機》 Convergence of Jade Mechanisms

héng 骱 lower leg

héng gé 橫格 horizontal block *(death pulse texture of gallbladder qi insufficiency)*

héng luò 衡絡 literally "balance network" or horizontal collateral, an alternate name for the Belt Vessel

héng nǔ 橫弩 crossbow

héng suān 骱酸 *calf soreness*

hóu 喉 pharynx

hòu 後 after, behind, euphemism for anus

hòu 候 wait, also a 5 day week

hóu bì 喉痹 *throat impediment*

hòu bú lì 後不利 *constipation*, literally "behind inhibited"

hòu xiè 後泄 *diarrhea*

hū 乎 particle, indicates exclamation point at end of sentence

hū 呼 exhalation, exclamation

hǔ 虎 tiger

hù 戶 singledoor

hū hū 忽忽 *frustratedly, fleetingly*

hú shàn 狐疝 *fox hernia* (Wiseman: foxlike mounting)

huá 華 magnificence *(death pulse texture of Small Intestine qi insufficiency)*

huá 滑 slippery

huà 化 transformation

Huà Tuó jiá jǐ 華佗夾脊 acupoints M-BW-35

huà wù 化物 transforming substance

huài 壞 bad, broken, ruin

huái zǐ 懷子 pregnancy

huǎn 緩 slow, moderate, (v.) to ease or make slower

huán tiào 環跳 Ring Jump, acupoint Gallbladder 30 (Wiseman: Jumping Round)

huáng dǎn 黃疸 *jaundice*

Huángdì Bāshíyī Nànjīng 《黃帝八十一難經》 The Yellow Emperor's Classic of 81 Difficulties

Huángdì Nèijīng 《黃帝內經》 The Yellow Emperor's Internal Classic

Huángdì Wàijīng 《黃帝外經》 The Yellow Emperor's External Classic

Huángfǔ Mì 皇甫謐 Eastern Han and Jin Dynasty scholar, author of Zhenjiu Jiayi Jing

huì yīn 會陰 Meeting Yin, acupoint Ren 1

hún 魂 ethereal soul

hūn huò 昏惑 *dementia* (Wiseman: confused and dazed)

huǒ 火 fire

huò 惑 confusion

huò 或 or

huò luàn 霍亂 *sudden chaos* (Wiseman: acute gastroenteritis, cholera, sudden turmoil)

huǒ zhú guāng yě 火燭光也 whatever happens when yang bìng-merges above, literally "fire candle light end-of-sentence"

jī 雞 chickens

jī 積 *accumulation*

jī 肌 muscle

jī 機 mechanism, also the side of the hip

jī 朞 one sixth of a zhōu-circuit of sky's qì-node, equal to one year

jí 極 utmost, extreme

jí 急 urgent, acute, hurried

jí 及 as well as

jí 瘠 emaciation and weakness

jǐ 己 6th heavenly stem

jǐ 脊 vertebrae, spine

jì 伎 skill, archaic term for a professional female dancer or singer

jì 紀 record, chronicle, document

jì 悸 *palpitations*

jī bì 肌痹 *muscle impediment*

jí duó 亟奪 *urgently taken by force* (Wiseman: urgent despoliation)

jī fū 肌膚 muscle and surface [fascia], i.e. inner part of the body's exterior

jī guān bú lì 機關不利 *joints inarticulate*, literally "hinges inhibited"

jí jiàng 脊強 *spinal stiffness* [of the Du Mai]

jī qì 積氣 *accumulation of qi*

jì qiǎo 伎巧 talent and agility (Wiseman: ingenuity)

jī ròu 肌肉 muscle and flesh

jī ròu rún suān 肌肉瞤酸 *muscle soreness*

jī ròu wěi 肌肉痿 *muscle atrophy*

jī ròu zhēn fā 肌肉胗發 *muscle pustule eruptions*

jī sōu xiě 積溲血 *accumulation hematuria*

jī xīn fù shí mǎn 積心腹時滿 *accumulation of heart and abdomen with periodic fullness*

jì xià 季夏 longsummer

jī yǐn 積飲 *accumulation rheum*

jǐ zhōng 脊中 Vertebrae Center, acupoint Du 6 (Wiseman: Spinal Center)

jiǎ 甲 1st heavenly stem

jiǎ 瘕 *conglomeration*

jiá chē 頰車 Cheek Cart, acupoint Stomach 6 (Wiseman: cheek carriage)

jiá zhǒng 頰腫 *cheeks swollen*

jiǎ jù 瘕聚 *conglomeration and gathering* [of the Ren Mai]

jiǎo 角 dragonhorn (*Chinese constellation*), also 3rd note on musical scale [roughly equivalent to Mi]

jiào 教 teaching(s)

jiǎo qī 交漆 filtering lacquer (*death pulse texture*)

jiǎo xià tòng 腳下痛 *foot/sole pain*

jiāo xìn 交信 Exchange Trust, acupoint Kidney 9 (Wiseman: Intersection Reach)

jiān 肩 shoulder

jiān 堅 harden, hard, firm

jiàn 見 to see, to meet, or to be exposed to

jiàn 楗 between fibula and pubic bones, literally "bolt"

jiān bèi rè 肩背熱 *shoulder/upper back heat*

jiān bèi tòng 肩背痛 *shoulder/upper back pain*

jiān chéng 堅成 hard accomplishment *(excess metal year name)*

jiān jiě 肩解 Shoulder Release, alternate acupoint name for Gallbladder 21 or Small Intestine 12

jiān jǐng 肩井 Shoulder Well, acupoint Gallbladder 21

jiān jué 煎厥 *boiling reversal*

jiān pǐ 堅否 *hard glomus*

jiān qì 間氣 between qi

jiān xià 堅下 *hard stools*

jiàn yì 諫議 discusser, one who uses direct speech and debate to change behavior

jiān zhēn 肩貞 Shoulder True, acupoint Small Intestine 9 (Wiseman: True Shoulder)

jiàng 降 descending

Jiǎng Lè 蔣樂 Amy's student at the Acupuncture and Integrative Medicine College (AIMC), Berkeley

jiàng jūn 將軍 general

jiàng pū 僵仆 *stiff syncope*

jiàng shàng 強上 *stiffness above*

jiē 皆 all

jiě 解 explanation

jié 節 rhythm, regularity, node, [musculoskeletal] joint, solar term, holiday, moderation, governance (Wiseman: regulation) jié 結 knot

jié jìng fǔ 潔淨府 promote urination, literally "clean the clean fu-organ"

jié luò 節絡 nodes [and] collaterals

jiĕ mài 解脈 Separator Vessel, i.e., a branch of the Foot Taiyang

jiē nuè 痎瘧 intermittent ague (Wiseman: agonizing torment disease, i.e. malaria)

jīn 筋 sinew, sinews

jīn 津 thin body fluids

jīn 今 now

jīn 金 metal

jīn 黔 golden-yellow

jǐn 謹 carefully, solemnly, sincerely

jìn 盡 terminate, eliminate, exhaust, finish

jìn 近 near, local, proximity

jìn 禁 taboo, forbidden

jīn bì 筋痹 sinew impediment

jìn cháo 晉朝 Jin Dynasty (265-420)

jīn chí 筋弛 sinew laxity

jīn gǔ 筋骨 sinews and bones

jīn gǔ bìng bì 筋骨併辟 sinews/bones split together?

jīn gǔ yáo fù 筋骨繇復 sinews/bones forced labor?

jīn guì 金匱 golden cabinet, strongbox, bookcase, safe

Jīn Guì Yào Luè 《金匱要略》 Essentials of the Golden Cabinet

jǐn hòu 謹候 to observe closely, literally "carefully/sincerely await"

jīn jí 筋急 sinew cramps

jīn lán zhī shì 金蘭之室 golden lotus room

jǐn liǎn 緊斂 tight restraint (transformation of metal)

jīn luán 筋攣 sinew cramps (Wiseman: hypertonicity of the sinews)

jìn qiè 勁切 forceful severance (governance of metal)

jīn wěi 筋痿 sinew atrophy (Wiseman: sinew wilting)

jīn yè 津液 body fluids

jìn yín 浸淫 immersion, i.e. infection

Jīnguì Yào Luè 《金匱要略》 Essentials from the Golden Cabinet, 2nd half of Shanghan Zabing Lun

jīng 精 essence

jīng 經 classic, channels/meridians, menses, longitude

jīng 驚 startled, shock (Wiseman: fright)

jǐng 井 well

jìng 靜 quiet, quietude

jìng 脛 shin

jìng 痙 convulsions

jīng míng 睛明 Eyeball Brightness, acupoint Bladder 1

jǐng dǐ zhī wā 井底之蛙 well bottom's frog (proverb)

jīng diǎn 經典 classical text

jīng hài 驚駭 shock terrors (Wiseman: fright, panic)

jīng huò 驚惑 shock-induced disorientation

jīng jì 經紀 channels and records

jīng kuáng 驚狂 shock mania (Wiseman: fright mania)

jīng luò 經絡 channels and collaterals

jīng mài 經脈 channels and vessels

jīng nǜ 驚衄 shock nosebleed

jīng shén 精神 essence and spirit, also modern term for psychology

jìng shùn 靜順 quiet submissive (even water year name)

jīng sōu bú lì 涇溲不利 inhibited urination

jīng suān 脛酸 shin soreness

jīng suì 經隧 channel tunnel

jīng wēi 精微 essence subtleties

jǐng yōng 頸癰 neck ulcer

jǐng xiàng tòng 頸項痛 neck [and] nape pain

jìng zhǒng 脛腫 shin swelling

jiǒng 炅 warmth, firelight

jiǒng zhōng 炅中 intense heat in middle [jiao]

jiǔ 九 nine

jiǔ 久 long, chronic, enduring

jiǔ 灸 moxibustion

jiù 就 to move toward

jiù 咎 disaster, bad fortune, woe

jiǔ bǐng 灸炳 moxibustion

jiǔ fēng 久風 chronic wind (Wiseman: enduring wind)

jiǔ fēng 酒風 alcohol wind

jiǔ hòu 九候 nine indicators (pulse positions)

jiǔ lì 久立 stand for long [period of time]

jiǔ qiào 九竅 nine orifices

jiū wěi 鳩尾 Turtledove Tail, acupoint Ren 15 (Wiseman: turtle-doves tail)

jiǔ zuò 久坐 sit for long [period of time]

jū 拘 constrict

jū 疽 abscess

jū 居 reside, dwell

jǔ 舉 raise, lift, adduct

jù 拒 reject

jù 俱 simultaneously

jù 聚 gather, gathering

jù cì 巨刺 contralateral-channel pricking (acupuncture technique), literally "giant pricking"

jù gǔ 巨骨 Giant Bone, acupoint name for Large Intestine 15 and also the clavicle

jū luán 拘攣 hypertonicity

jū qì 居氣 resident qi

jū shì 居室 to reside indoors

jù xū 巨虛 Giant Hollow, alternate acupoint name of Stomach 37 & 39 [usually implies St37 unless specified as "lower"]

jù yáng 巨陽 alternate name for taiyang, literally "giant yang"

juǎn 卷 curl

jué 厥 *reversal*

jué 決 to decide or be decisive, to breach a dam

jué 絕 to terminate, end, vanish

jué dú 決瀆 irrigation (Wiseman: keep the sluices clear)

jué duàn 決斷 judgment and decisions (Wiseman: resolution, decisiveness)

jué nì 厥逆 *reversal counterflow* (Wiseman: reversal flow)

jué shàn 厥疝 *reversal hernia* (Wiseman: reversal mounting)

juéyīn 厥陰 terminal yin

jūn 君 emperor [herb]

jūn héng 均衡 equal level, or equilibrium *(transformation of even fire year)*

jūn zhǔ 君主 emperor (Wiseman: monarch, sovereign)

jūn zǐ 君子 "gentleman" AKA a person of character

kāi 開 to open

kài 欬 archaic character for cough <Amy: I use this character throughout the text instead of 咳>

kǎi bèi 豈備 triumphant preparation *(transformation of earth)*

kāi guǐ mén 開鬼門 induce sweating, literally "open ghost doors"

kāng 康 health

kàng 亢 dragonthroat *(Chinese constellation)*

kāo 尻 sacrum

kāo yīn gǔ xī bì chuǎn héng jiē bìng 尻陰股膝髀腨胻足皆病 *Sacrum, Genital, Buttock, Knee, Hip, Calf, Shin and Leg Disease*

ké 咳 cough <Amy: I use the archaic character 欬 in this text>

ké 殼 shell

kě 渴 thirst

kě 可 can

kè 刻 quarter of an hour

kě ér chuān jǐng 「渴而穿井」 dig well when thirsty *(proverb)*

kè qì 客氣 guest qi

ké sòu 咳嗽 cough <Note from Amy: this is the modern word-phrase we use today.>

kè zhǔ rén 客主人 Guest Master, literally "guest, host-human", alternate acupoint name for Gallbladder 3

kōng 空 space, emptiness

kǒng 恐 fear

Kǒng-fūzǐ 孔夫子 Confucius, literally "Master Kong"

Kǒng Qiū 孔丘 Confucius' actual name

kǒng rú rén jiāng bǔ zhī 恐如人將捕之 *fearful as if about to be arrested*, i.e. paranoid

kǒu 口 mouth

kǒu chuāng 口瘡 *mouth ulcer*

kǒu gān 口乾 *dry mouth*

kǒu mí 口糜 *oral putrefaction*

kǔ 苦 bitter

kuài rán 快然 feel good, gratified

kuān 髖 hip

kuān bì rú bié 髖髀如別 *hip and thigh [feel] as if separated*

kuáng 狂 *mania*

kuáng yuè 狂越 *manic boundary-crossing*

kuí 奎 tigerlegs *(Chinese constellation)*

Kuí Duó 《揆度》 Formulas and Pulses

lán 蘭 orchid

Lán Shì 蘭室 Orchid Chamber, the Emperor's Imperial Library

láo 醪 undecanted wine with dregs

láo 勞 exertion (Wiseman: taxation)

láo fēng 勞風 *taxation wind*

láo lǐ 醪醴 medicinal wines, alcoholic infusions

lèi 類 category, categories

Léi Gōng 雷公 Thunder Duke, name of Yellow Emperor's student

lěng 冷 cold [in an object or body part]

lí 離 separation, departure, also the trigram for fire

lǐ 裡 interior

lǐ 理 reason, order, also short for geography

lǐ 醴 sweet wine, medicinal liquor

lǐ 里 unit of distance equivalent to one third of a mile

lì 利 (adj.) sharp, uninhibited, also (v.) to benefit

lì 癘 *pestilence*

lì 立 stand, also short for 立刻 (lì kè) "immediately"

lì chūn 立春 start of spring *(solar term)*

lì duì 歷兌 Experienced Marsh[-trigram], acupoint Stomach 25 (Wiseman: severe mouth)

lì fēng 癘風 *pestilential wind*

Lǐ Guóqīng 李國清 contemporary Neijing annotator

lǐ jí 裡急 *tenesmus*

lì liè 溧冽 shivering cold *(change of water)*

liǎn 斂 restrained

liáng 涼 cool

liǎng 兩 bilateral, pair

liǎng bì nèi tòng 兩臂內痛 *bilateral medial arm pain*

liǎng xié mǎn 兩脇滿 *bilateral rib fullness*

liǎng xié tòng 兩脇痛 *bilateral rib pain*

liǎng xié xià shào fù tòng 兩脇下少腹痛 bilateral rib/hypochondriac/hypogastric pain

liè 裂 crack

lín 臨 approach

lín 凜 shudder

lín bì 淋閟 *painful urine retention*

lín kuì 霖潰 continuous rain [and] rupture [as of breaking dams] *(catastrophe of earth)*

líng 靈 soul, magic

lìng 令 to express command(s), to cause

líng lán zhī shì 靈蘭之室 Chamber of Soul Orchids

líng shì 靈室 Soul Chamber, nickname for the Chamber of Soul Orchids

Líng Tái 靈臺 Soul Bier, the name of an observatory, acupoint Du 10 (Wiseman: spirit tower)

Língshū 《靈樞》 Magic Pivots, 2nd half of the Huangdi Neijing

liū 溜 slide *(pulse texture)*

liú 留 retain, keep, also food stagnation

liú 流 water moving

liǔ 柳 willowbeak *(Chinese constellation)*

liù 六 six

liù fǔ 六府 six Fu Organs (Unschuld: six palaces)

liù qì 六氣 six climatic factors

liú shuǐ 流水 *watery exudation*

Liú Wēnshū 劉溫舒 Song Dynasty Chinese medical practitioner, suspected author of Suwen 72-73

liú xiè jìn zhǐ 流泄禁止 *incontinence?* Literally "flow leak forbidden pause"

liú yǎn 流衍 flow superfluous *(excess water year name)*

liù yuán 六元 six origins

lóng 隆 swell, bulge, become abundant

lóng 聾 deaf

lóng 癃 *[urinary] dribbling or retention* (Wiseman: dribbling block)

lóng bì 癃閉 *urinary retention/blockage*

lóu 婁 garment-train *(Chinese constellation)*

lòu bìng 漏病 *leaking disease*

lòu fēng 漏風 *leaking wind*

lù 露 dew

lǚ (月呂) backbone <Note from Amy: this character is so archaic my computer cannot type it!>

lǜ (v.) 慮 to consider carefully; (n.) excessive thought, preoccupation

lǜ jiǎ 慮瘕 *anxiety conglomeration*

lǚ jīn 膂筋 paravertebral sinews

lǚ rú 蘆茹 alternate name for (qiàn cǎo gēn) 茜草根 madder root *(herb)*

lù xián cǎo 鹿銜草 pyrola *(herb)*

luán 攣 cramps

lùn 論 discussion

luàn 亂 chaos, disorder, revolution

luàn jīng 亂經 disrupted channels, occurs when erroneously treated during moon waning

luò 絡 collateral, connect, network, fiber

luò shū 絡俞 network points

mà lì 罵詈 curse, scold

Mǎ Shì 馬蒔 (1400s-1500s, exact birth/death dates unknown) Míng Dynasty 明朝 (1368–1644) royal physician, first person to annotate the Língshū

mài 脈 [blood] vessel(s), pulse

mài bì 脈痹 *vessel impediment*

Mài Fǎ 《脈法》 Pulse Method

mài fēng 脈風 *vessel wind*

Mài Jīng 《脈經》 Pulse Classic

mài wěi 脈痿 *vessel atrophy* (Wiseman: vessel wilting)

mài yào 脈要 pulse essentials

mǎn 滿 fullness, full [of energy]

máo 毛 fur, i.e. body hair; feather *(pulse texture)*

mǎo 卯 4th earthly branch, 5-7am, 3/6-4/4, year of the Rabbit, spring equinox, compass point 90°, east

mǎo 昴 tigerfuzz *(Chinese constellation)*

mào chóng 瞀重 *diplopia*, literally "visual distortion doubled"

mào wèi 瞀昧 *blurry vision/taste*

mào yù 瞀鬱 *malaise with dizziness*

mén 門 doors, gates

mén hù 門戶 doors and windows

méng mèi 蒙昧 *blurry vision*

miàn 面 face

miàn chì 面赤 *face red*

miàn hēi 面黑 *face black*

miàn sè 面色 complexion, literally "face color"

miào hū zāi wèn yě 「妙乎哉問也」'Excellent question!'

miè 滅 to extinguish

mín 民 people

mǐn 敏 agility

míng 明 (adj.) bright, (v.) to clarify or brighten

mìng 命 life, fate, lifespan

míng cháo 明朝 Ming Dynasty (1368-1644)

mìng mén 命門 Life Gate, acupoint Du 4, alternate acupoint name for Bladder 1

mìng qì 命氣 life qi

míng yào 明曜 bright illumination *(governance of fire)*

miù cì 繆刺 contralateral-collateral pricking *(acupuncture technique)*

mó 摩 scoured

mò 沫 foam

mò shì 末世 (Wiseman: last phase of an age)

mò zhī qí jí 莫知其極 not know its extreme

móu 謀 strategy, plan, scheme

móu lǜ 謀慮 deliberation; strategy and planning

mǔ 母 mother

mù 暮 dusk, sunset

mù 木 wood

mù bù míng 目不明 *eyes not bright*, i.e. poor vision

mù chì tòng 目赤痛 *eyes red [and] painful*

mù máng máng wú suǒ jiàn 目眈眈無所見 *vision blacks out*

mù fēng 目風 *eye wind*

mù míng 目冥 *blurry vision*

mù shì 暮世 twilight era, i.e. contemporary times

mù shì máng máng 目視眈眈 *blurry vision*

mù tòng 目痛 *eye pain*

mù wú suǒ jiàn 目無所見 *blindness*

mù zhī shuǐ 目之水 "water of the eyes", i.e. tears

nǎi 乃 participle that can mean so, therefore, or to be

nài hé 奈何 meaning what? (Wiseman: how?)

nào 淖 mud

nǎo fēng 腦風 *brain wind*

nǎo hù 腦戶 Brain Window, acupoint Du 17

nǎo shèn 腦滲 brain seepage

nào yè 淖液 liquid

nán 南 south

nán fēng 南風 south wind

nán miàn 南面 south facing

nán zǐ 男子 men

Nàn Jīng 《難經》 Classic of Difficulties, nickname of the Huangdi Bashiyi Nan Jing

nánběi cháo 南北朝 Nanbei Dynasty, literally "Southern and Northern Dynasties" (420-589)

nèi 內 inner, inside

nèi duó 內奪 *internal robbery*?

nèi fēng 內風 *internal wind*

nèi jié 內結 *internal knots* [disease of the Ren Mai]

nèi rè 內熱 internal heat

nèi zhēn 內鍼 insert needle

Nèijīng 《內經》 Internal Classic, nickname of the Huangdi Neijing

néng 能 can, able to, (n.) capability

ní 泥 mud, muddy

nì 匿 concealed, anonymous

nì 逆 counterflow, rebellious

nì qì 逆氣 *counterflow qi* [disease of the Chong Mai]

niào chì 溺赤 *red urine*

niào xiě 溺血 *hematuria* (Wiseman: bloody urine)

níng 寧 tranquility

níng 凝 congeal

níng qì 凝泣 coagulate

níng sù 凝肅 congeal solemnity *(governance of water)*

niú 牛 Cowherd, short for (niú láng) 牛郎 "cow[herding] youth" *(Chinese constellation)*

nóng fū 膿腑 *pus rot*

nǚ 女 Weavergirl, short for (zhī nǚ) 織女 "weaving woman" *(Chinese constellation)*

nǜ 衄 nosebleed, i.e. epistaxis

nù 怒 anger

nǜ miè 衄衊 *nosebleed*, i.e. epistaxis

nǜ miè míng mù 衄衊瞑目 *fatal nosebleed*

nǚ zǐ 女子 women

nuè 瘧 *ague* (Wiseman: malaria)

ǒu 嘔 retch, retching

ǒu xiě 嘔血 *retch blood*, i.e. hematemesis

ǒu xiè 嘔泄 *retching diarrhea*

ǒu yǒng 嘔涌 *reflux*

páng 傍 beside

páng guāng 膀胱 urinary bladder

pèi lán 佩蘭 eupatorium *(herb)*

pí 皮 skin

pí 脾 spleen

pǐ 否 hexagram 8 from the I Ching, glomus <Note from Amy: later texts use the character 痞 (pǐ) with the disease radical.>

pì 癖 *blockage*, short for *intestinal blockage* 腸癖 (cháng pì)

pì 譬 for example

pí bì 皮痹 *skin impediment*

pí bì 脾痹 *spleen impediment*

pí bù 皮部 skin area(s)

pí dān 脾癉 *spleen drought* (Wiseman: splenic pure heat)

pí fēng 脾風 *spleen wind*, alternate disease/pattern name for dān 癉 *drought*

pí fēng shàn 肺風疝 *spleen wind hernia*

pí fū 皮膚 skin and surface

pí máo 皮毛 skin and pores, outermost surface of body

pì jī 癖積 *aggregation*

pí xū 脾虛 spleen deficiency

pì yīn 辟陰 *split yin*

piān fēng 偏風 *asymmetrical wind* (Wiseman: hemilateral wind)

piān kū 偏枯 *asymmetrical withering* (Wiseman: hemiplegia)

piān sāi 偏塞 *asymmetrical congestion*

piān xū 偏虛 *asymmetrical deficiency*

pǐn 品 class, grade, rankings

píng 平 flat, i.e. balanced

píng 評 evaluation, critique

píng dàn 平旦 daybreak

píng qì 平氣 even qi

píng rén 平人 balanced person

pò 魄 corporeal soul

pò 迫 press, compel, force (Wiseman: distress)

pò mén 魄門 gate of po, i.e. anus

pū 仆 to fall forward, i.e. faint

pū jí 仆擊 *syncope*

qī 七 seven

qí 其 classical Chinese all-purpose pronoun

qǐ 起 rise, get up, initiate [action]

qí 齊 simultaneously, evenly

qí 奇 extraordinary

qì 氣 air, breath, vital energy, weather, season, flatulence, solar term

qì 泣 *coagulation*, also tears

Qí Bó 岐伯 name of Huangdi's royal physician

qì bìng 氣并 qi merge

qì bù tōng 氣不通 qì stagnation, literally "qi no throughput"

qì chōng 氣衝 Qi Rushing, acupoint Stomach 30, where the Chōng Mài begins (Wiseman: qi thoroughfare)

qì chū 泣出 tearing [of the eyes]

qí cì 其次 secondly, next

Qí Héng 《奇恆》 Extraordinary Prognoses

qí héng zhī fǔ 奇恆之府 the extraordinary Fu-organs

qì huà 氣化 qi transformation

qì jiāo 氣交 qi exchange

Qì Jiāo Biàn 《氣交變》 Qi Exchange Changes

qì jiē 氣街 Qi Street, alternate acupoint name for Stomach 30

qì jué 氣絕 stop breathing, i.e. die

qì jué 氣厥 *qi reversal*

qì kǒu 氣口 the radial pulse, literally "qi mouth"

qì mǎn 氣滿 *qi fullness*

qì mǎn fā nì 氣滿發逆 *qi fullness expressing [as] counterflow*

qì nì 氣逆 *qi counterflow*

qì pò 氣迫 qi oppressed, the deficiency of not arriving by the proper time

qī shàn 七疝 *seven hernias* [disease of the Ren Mai] (Wiseman: seven mountings)

qì shàng 氣上 *qi ascension*

qì xiàng 氣象 qi and appearance, i.e. aura; modern day term for atmosphere

qí xiū 齊脩 simultaneous cultivation *(transformation of even earth year)*

qì xué 氣穴 qi cave

qī yào 七曜 seven shining celestial bodies, i.e. the sun, the moon, Venus, Jupiter, Mercury, Mars, and Saturn

qì yī 棄衣 abandon garments

qì yín 氣淫 qi excess, the overacting of arriving before the proper time

qián 前 front, euphemism for urethra

qián 錢 unit of weight approximately equal to 3.75g

qiǎn 淺 shallow, superficial

qiàn 欠 yawn

qián bì 前閉 *frontal block*, i.e. urinary blockage

qiàn cǎo gēn 茜草根 modern herb name for madder root

qiáng 強 strong

qiǎo 巧 cleverness, agility, workmanship

qiào 竅 orifice

qiào yīn 竅陰 Orifice Yin, acupoint Gallbladder 44

qiě 且 also

qiè rán 怯然 *fearfulness* (Wiseman: timidity)

qǐn hàn 寢汗 *night sweats*, "sweating in bed"

qīng 清 clear, clarity; archaic term for cool

qíng 情 situation, feeling (Wiseman: affect)

qīng jié 清潔 cool [and] clean (virtue of metal)

qīng jué 清厥 *cool reversal*, i.e. cold feet

qīng mì 清謐 clear tranquility (transformation of water)

qiū 秋 autumn (season)

qiú 鼽 *nasal congestion* (Wiseman: sniveling)

qiú 求 to plead, to beg

qiú gǔ 鼽骨 nasal congestion bone, i.e. zygoma?

qiú nǜ 鼽衄 *nasal congestion [with] nosebleed*

qiú tì 鼽嚏 *nasal congestion [with] sneezing*

qiū xíng 秋刑 the punishment of fall

qū 曲 to flex [a muscle or limb]

qū 胠 archaic term for torso from waist to armpits

qū 傴 humpback

qǔ 取 to take

qù 去 go, remove, eliminate, subtract

qū bù néng shēn 曲不能伸 flexion without extension

qù gù 去故 let go of the past

qū shēn bú lì 屈伸不利 difficulty flexing/extending

quán 全 (adj.) whole, complete, (v.) to integrate

Quán Yuánqǐ 全元起 scholar of the Nanbei Dynasty whose annotation of the Neijing was referenced by Wang Bing

quē 缺 to wane, lack, make less complete

quē pén 缺盆 Chipped Basin, acupoint Stomach 12, also the name of the supraclavicular fossa (Wiseman: empty basin)

rǎo 擾 disturb, bother

rè 熱 heat

rè bì 熱痹 *heat impediment*

rè jué 熱厥 *heat reversal*

rè zhì 熱至 heat arrival, i.e. pathogenic heat arrives during hot weather

rè zhòng 熱中 *heat stroke*

rén 人 human(s), people

rèn 任 control <Amy: often mistranslated as (rèn) 妊 "conception" of the same pronunciation>

rèn 壬 9th heavenly stem

rèn mài 任脈 Controlling Vessel

rén yíng 人迎 Human Welcome, acupoint Stomach 9 and also the carotid pulse (Wiseman: mans prognosis)

rì 日 day, sun, date

rì mù 日暮 sunset, dusk

rì xī 日西 afternoon

rì zhōng 日中 midday, i.e. noon

róng 容 (v.) to absorb, accept, contain; (n.) countenance

róng 榮 glory, luxuriance, sometimes stands in for (yíng) 營 "nutritive/construction"

róng píng 容平 contain [and] balance, or tolerate [and] suppress

róng qì 榮氣 alternate characters for nutritive/(yíng qì) 營氣 "construction qi"

róng wèi 榮衛 construction/defensive [qi]

róu 柔 soft, soften

ròu 肉 flesh

ròu bì 肉痹 *flesh impediment*

róu jìng 柔痙 *soft tetany*

ròu lǐ 肉里 flesh lining <Wang Bing: related to the Shaoyang and Yangwei>

ròu rún chì 肉膶瘲 *muscle twitches/convulsions*

ròu tòng 肉痛 *muscle pain*, i.e. myalgia

ròu wěi 肉痿 *flesh atrophy* (Wiseman: flesh wilting)

rú 如 as if

rú 濡 immersion, soggy, pith? juice?

rù 入 enter

rù 溽 damp summerheat

rú huǒ xīn rán 如火薪然 like fire catching (*death pulse texture of heart essence being robbed*)

rú xiè 濡泄 *soggy diarrhea*

rù zhēng 溽蒸 humid steam (*virtue of earth*)

ruǎn 耎 to soften or make more flexible

ruǎn lì 緛戾 *gnarled cramps*

rún 瞤 *[eye] twitch*

rùn 潤 moisten

rún chì 膶瘲 *[muscle] twitches/convulsions*

ruò 若 as if

ruò suǒ ài zài wài 「若所愛在外」 'as if [that which is] beloved is outside'

sǎ sǎ zhèn hán 洒洒振寒 endless shivering chills

sāi 塞 congestion or to congest, literally "stopper"

sān 三 three

sǎn 散 powder (herbs) <Wang Bing: also a branch of the Spleen Channel>

sàn 散 scattered, (v.) to disperse/scatter

sān bù 三部 three parts *(pulse positions)*

sān lǐ 三里 Three Miles, acupoint Stomach 36 Foot Three Miles and Large Intestine 10 Hand Three Miles

sān rì 三日 three days

sǎn shū 散俞 scattered points <Unschuld: ashi points scattered along the channel>

sàn luò 散落 scatter [and] fall/drop (*catastrophe of wood*)

sàn yè 散葉 scattered leaves (*death pulse texture of liver qi deficiency*)

sè 色 color, complexion

sè 濇 grating, rough, choppy

sè sè 色色 all kinds

shā 殺 (v.) to kill, (n.) killing

shàn 善 adept/good at, tendency for, also an affirmative sound

shàn 疝 hernia, pathological protrusion (Wiseman: mounting)

shàn bēi 善悲 *tendency for sadness*, i.e. melancholy

shàn chì 善瘛 *tendency to cramp*

shàn jiǎ 疝瘕 *hernia conglomeration* (Wiseman: mounting-conglomeration)

shàn kǒng 善恐 *tendency for fearfulness*, i.e. timidity

shàn nù 善怒 *tendency for anger*, i.e. irritability

shàn tài xī 善太息 *tendency to sigh*, i.e. frequent sighing

shàn wàng 善忘 *tendency to forget*, i.e. forgetfulness

shāng 傷 damage, injure, harm

shāng 商 2nd note on musical scale, roughly equivalent to Re

shàng 上 high, top, above, rise

shàng 尚 yet

shàng chǐ hán 上齒寒 *upper teeth cold*

shàng chuǎn 上喘 *upper panting*

shàng dì 上帝 high emperor

shàng gōng 上工 superior practitioner(s)

shàng guān 上關 Upper Gate, acupoint Gallbladder 3

shāng hán 傷寒 *cold damage*

shàng jì 上紀 Upper Record, alternate acupoint name for Ren 12

Shàng Jīng 《上經》 Upper Classic

shàng jù xū 上巨虛 Upper Giant Hollow, acupoint Stomach 37

shàng qì 上氣 *hyperventilation?*

shāng shí 傷食 *food damage*

shāng shǔ 傷暑 *summerheat damage*

shàng wǎn 上脘 Upper Abdominal-Cavity, acupoint Ren 13

shàng xià bù tōng 上下不通 *inhibition above and below* (Wiseman: stoppage high and low)

shàng xià sān pǐn 上下三品 superior-inferior 3 [herb] categories

shàng xià zhōng hán 上下中寒 *upper lower middle cold*

shàn xū xià shí 上虛下實 *empty above [and] solid below*

Shānghán Zábìng Lùn 《傷寒雜病論》 Discussion on Cold Damage and Miscellaneous Diseases

Shānghán Lùn 《傷寒論》 Discussion on Cold Damage, 1st half of Shanghan Zabing Lun

shǎo 少 scant, few, less, minus

shào 少 lesser, younger

shào fù 少腹 lower abdomen [area below navel], i.e. hypogastrium (Wiseman: lesser abdomen)

shào fù tòng 少腹痛 *lower abdominal pain*, i.e. hypogastric pain

shào fù yuān rè 少腹冤熱 *hypogastric veiling heat*

shào fù zhǒng 少腹腫 *hypogastric swelling*

shǎo qì 少氣 *scant qi*, i.e. shortness of breath (Wiseman: scantness of breath)

shǎo qì zhī jué 少氣之厥 *reversal of scant qi*

shǎo xiě 少血 *scant blood*, i.e. anemia

shàoyáng 少陽 lesser yang

shàoyīn 少陰 lesser yin

shé 舌 tongue

shé juǎn 舌卷 *tongue curled*, i.e. aphasia

shé juǎn bù néng yán 舌卷不能言 *[motor] aphasia*

shēn 深 deep

shēn 身 body [especially the torso: shoulder, spine, sacrum]

shēn 申 9th earthly branch, 3-5pm, 8/7-9/7, year of the Monkey, compass point 240°

shēn 伸 extension

shén 神 spirit, spirits, God

shèn 腎 kidney

shèn 甚 extreme (Wiseman: severe)

shèn bì 腎痹 *kidney impediment*

shèn fēng shàn 腎風疝 *kidney wind hernia*

shēn mài 申脈 Extending Vessel, acupoint Bladder 62

shén mén 神門 Spirit Door, acupoint Heart 7

shén míng 神明 spirit and brightness, divinity, gods (Wiseman: bright spirit)

shén píng 審平 (*even metal year name*)

shén què 神闕 Spirit Gate-Tower, acupoint Ren 8

shēn rè 身熱 *body hot*

shēn (tǐ) zhòng 身(體)重 *body heavy*

shēn tòng 身痛 *body pain*

shèn xū 腎虛 kidney deficiency

shén yòng wú fāng 神用無方 spirit function cannot be formulated

shēn yuān 深淵 deep abyss

shēng 生 to create, generate, give birth to

shēng 升 ascending, also a unit of volume equal to approximately 200 milliliters

shěng 眚 calamity

shèng 勝 to win, defeat, triumph [over], get the better of, i.e. control/overact

shèng 盛 abundant

shēng dì huáng 生地黃 raw rehmannia root *(herb)*

shēng míng 升明 upbear brightness *(even fire year name)*

shèng (rén) 聖(人) the "sage" or sacred person

shēng róng 生榮 generate glory *(transformation of wood)*

shèng shuāi 盛衰 abundance and decline

shèng shuǐ 盛水 abundant water, i.e. time of year when ice and snow melts

shēng tiě luò 生鐵洛 iron flakes, Ferri Frusta

Shénnóng 神農 the Divine Husbandman

Shénnóng Běncǎo Jīng 《神農本草經》 Divine Husbandman's Materia Medica

shī 濕 damp, wet

shī 失 lose

shí 石 stone *(pulse texture)*, also short for bloodletting biǎn stones

shí 時 season of six solar terms, i.e. 90 days, can also mean periodic or occasional

shí 十 ten

shí 實 (adj.) solid [with tangible substance], excess (Wiseman: replete, repletion, replenish), (v.) to supplement (Wiseman: to firm)

shí 食 (v.) to eat

shí 蝕 eclipse, to erode

shǐ 始 (n.) beginning, origin (v.) to begin

shǐ 使 envoy [herb] (Wiseman: courier); (v.) cause to be

shì 市 market

shì 室 room *(Chinese constellation)*

shì 視 view, look at

shì 示 indication(s), sign, revelation

shí bì 食痹 *food impediment*

shí bú huà 食不化 indigestion (Wiseman: non-transformation of food)

shí chòu 食臭 the smell of food, literally "food stench"

shī dào 失道 losing the Way

shí èr 十二 12

shí èr jīng mài 十二經脈 12 channels and vessels

shì gù 是故 therefore

shī guǐ 屍鬼 corpse ghost(s)

shí jiǎn 食減 *reduced appetite*

shī jīng 失精 *loss of essence*

shí jīng 時驚 *periodic shock*

shī jué 屍厥 *corpse reversal* (Wiseman: deathlike reversal)

shí shǎo 食少 *reduced food intake*, literally "food less"

shī shǒu 失守 lose guard

shí shuǐ 石水 *stone water*, also perhaps the time of year when water freezes hard as stone

shī wèi 失味 *loss of taste*

shí yī 十一 11

shì yǐ 是以 therefore

shí yì 食亦 *food changes*

shí yǐn bú xià 食飲不下 *inability to eat or drink*

shí zé ǒu 食則嘔 *postprandial retching*, literally "food then retch"

shī zhěn 失枕 *losing pillow*, i.e. acute torticollis

shōu 收 withdraw, collect, absorb, contract, astringe

shǒu 手 hand

shǒu bù jí tóu 手不及頭 *hand cannot reach head*

shǒu fēng 首風 *head wind*

shōu liǎn 收斂 withdraw and restrain

shòu shèng 受盛 sorter, literally "receiving abundance" (Wiseman: reception and holding)

shǒu xīn zhǔ 手心主 Hand Heart Master, alternate name of Hand Jueyin Pericardium

shǒu zú hán 手足寒 *hands and feet cold*

shū 俞 acupoint, also a hollow boat made of bamboo i.e. canoe; the Neijing uses this character for both back-shu, shu-stream, and general acupoints

shū 輸 more modern character for shu-stream transport point

shū 樞 pivot

shū 疏 to neglect, also to dredge

shǔ 暑 summerheat, implies dampness/humidity

shǔ 黍 glutinous millet

shù 數 rapid, number, numbers

shǔ bìng 暑病 *summerheat disease*

shū chí 樞持 pivot-holder, yang of shaoyang skin area

shù gǔ 束骨 Bundle Bone, acupoint Bladder 65

shǔ lóu 鼠瘻 *mouse fistula*

shǔ shǔ 蜀黍 sorghum

Shuōwén Jiězì 《說文解字》 Explicating Words, Explaining Characters, the

2nd oldest dictionary of Chinese which back to the 2nd Century

shū qǐ 舒啟 stretch [and] open *(governance of wood)*

shū qiào 俞竅 deep points, literally "acupoint orifices"

shù rì 數日 several days

shū rú 樞儒 pivot scholar *(yin of shaoyin skin area)*

shù wèn 數問 ask several times

shū zhōng 樞中 Pivot Center, alternate acupoint name for Gallbladder 30

shū zhōng tòng 樞中痛 Gallbladder 30 pain, i.e. hip or piriformis pain

shuāi 衰 frail

shuàn yuān 腨痟 *calf weakness*

shuǐ 水 water, or radical 氵 (3 drops on the left side of characters), sometimes shorthand for edema

shuǐ dào 水道 waterways

shuǐ gǔ 水穀 water and grains, i.e. diet

shuǐ qì 水氣 *water qi*

shuǐ xià 水下 <Amy: I think this is unit measurement of time but I could not find any definitions!>

shuò 朔 new moon

shuò huì 朔晦 new moon gloom

shùn 順 submissive, with the flow

sī 思 thought

sǐ 死 (v.) to die, (n.) death

sì 四 four

sì 巳 6th earthly branch, 9-11am, 5/5-6/5, year of the Snake, compass point 150°

sì bái 四白 Four White, acupoint Stomach 2, also the sclera

sǐ bú zhì 死不治 fatal, literally "death, not treatable"

sǐ bú kě zhì 死不可治 fatal, literally "death, cannot be treated"

sì dé 四德 four virtues

sì jūn zǐ tāng 四君子湯 Four Gentlemen's Decoction

sī qì 司氣 dominant qi

sì qì 四氣 "four qi", the four seasons

sì shī 四失 four losses

sì shí 四時 "four times", the four seasons

sī suì 司歲 dominant year(s)

sī tiān 司天 Controlling Heaven, indication of sky qi, i.e. first half of year *(six climatic factor terminology)*, also alternate acupoint name for Stomach 24

sì wéi 四維 four ordinal directions (NE, NW, SE, SW)

sī yì 私意 private thoughts/intentions, i.e. secrets

sì zhī 四肢 four limbs

sì zhī bù jǔ 四肢不舉 *inability to lift the limbs*

sì zhī bú yòng 四肢不用 *four limbs atrophy*

sì zhī xiè duò 四支解憜 *four limbs fatigue*

sòng cháo 宋朝 Song Dynasty (960-1279)

sù 素 (adj.) plain, white, (adv.) usually/habitually

sù 速 speedy

sù 肅 [serious and respectful] silence

sù shā 肅殺 silent killing *(change of metal)*

suān 酸 sour, also used to indicate muscle soreness

suí 隨 follow, vary according to

suì 歲 year, one fifth of a zhōu-circuit of land's jì-record

suí kǒng 髓空 Marrow Space, alternate acupoint name for Du 2

suǒ 所 particle introducing a relative clause

suǒ wèi 所謂 what is called

suǒ zé 索澤 *rope marsh*

sūn luò 孫絡 grandchildren collaterals, i.e. capillaries

sūn xiè 飧泄 *lienteric diarrhea* (Wiseman: food diarrhea)

Sùwèn 《素問》 Plain Questions, 1st half of Huangdi Neijing

tái 台 platform

tài 太 greater

tāi bìng 胎病 *congenital seizures*

tài chōng 太沖 Great Rushing, acupoint Liver 3 (Wiseman: supreme surge)

tài guò 太過 too far past, overreaching, i.e. excess

tài xī 太溪 Great Stream, acupoint Kidney 3

tài xī 太息 sigh, literally "great respiration"

tài xū 太虛 great void, the cosmos

tài yuān 太淵 Great Abyss, acupoint Lung 9

Tàishǐ Tiānyuán Cè 《太史天元冊》 Book of Most Historical Sky Origins

tàiyáng 太陽 greater yang

tàiyīn 太陰 greater yin

tāng 湯 decoction, literally "soup"

táng 溏 loose stools

táng cháo 唐朝 Tang Dynasty (618-907)

táng xiè 溏泄 loose stools/diarrhea

tāng yè 湯液 water decoction

tǐ 體 body, divided into 12 parts (head: nape, face, cheeks; torso: shoulder, spine, sacrum; hand: upper arm, lower arm, hand; foot: thigh, calf, foot) according to the SWJZ

tì 嚏 *sneeze, sneezes, sneezing*

tì 涕 snot

tì rán 惕然 suddenly [fearful]

tǐ tòng 體痛 *body pain*

tǐ zhòng 體重 *body heaviness*

tiáo 調 to regulate or adjust

tiān 天 sky, heaven, weather, astrology

tiān chuāng 天窗 Sky Window, acupoint Small Intestine 16 (Wiseman: Celestial Window)

tiān (zhī) dào 天(之)道 heaven's way, i.e. natural law

tiān dì 天地 sky [and] land, i.e. between heaven and earth, in the world

tiān fǔ 天府 Sky Mansion, acupoint Lung 3 (Wiseman: Celestial Storehouse)

tiān gān 天干 [10] heavenly stems

tiān guǐ 天癸 skywater, the energetic substance that creates menses in female bodies and seminal emissions in male bodies; literally "sky 10th-heavenly-stem" (Wiseman: heavenly tenth, menses)

tiān qì 天氣 sky qi, i.e. weather

tiān shī 天師 Sky Master, a title for Qi Bo

tiān shū 天樞 Sky Pivot, acupoint Stomach 25

tiān tú 天突 Sky Protrusion, acupoint Ren 22 (Wiseman: Celestial Chimney)

tiān wén 天文 astronomy

tiān yǒu 天牖 Sky Wall-Window, acupoint Sanjiao 16 (Wiseman: Celestial Window)

tiān yuán jì 天元紀 sky origin records

tiān zhù 天柱 Sky Pillar, acupoint Bladder 10 (Wiseman: Celestial Pillar)

tīng 聽 to listen

tīng gōng 聽宮 Listening Palace, acupoint Small Intestine 19 (Wiseman: Auditory Palace)

tōng 通 throughput

tòng 痛 pain

tòng bì 痛痹 *painful impediment*

tóng bìng yì zhì 「同病異治」 'same disease, different treatment'

tòng jí xià lì 痛急下利 *painful/urgent diarrhea*

tōng píng 通評 complete evaluation

tóng yīn 同陰 Same Yin, i.e. a branch of the Foot Shaoyang

tòng yǐn shào fù 痛引少腹 *pain radiating to hypogastrium*

tóu 頭 head

tóu mù xuàn 頭目眩 *vertigo*

tóu nǎo hù tòng 頭腦戶痛 *head/Du17 pain*

tóu tòng 頭痛 *headache*

tóu xiàng jiān tòng 頭項肩痛 *head/nape/ shoulder pain*

tóu xiàng tòng 頭項痛 *head/nape pain*

tóu zhòng 頭重 *head heavy*

tǔ 土 earth

tù 吐 *vomit*

tù xià 吐下 *vomiting and diarrhea*

tuí 癀 erosion (Wiseman: slumping)

tuí shàn 癀疝 *genital hernia* (Wiseman: slumping mounting)

tuí tǔ 癀土 *ruined earth* (*death pulse texture of muscle qi insufficiency*)

tūn 吞 swallow

tuō 脫 desertion

tuò 唾 spittle

tuō xiě 脫血 *desertion of blood*

tuò xiě 唾血 *hemoptysis* (Wiseman: spitting of blood)

tuō yíng 脫營 *desertion of nourishment*

Urine Retentive Genital Hernia (tuí lóng shàn) 癀癃疝

wài 外 outer, outside

wài nèi 外內 outside and inside

wán 玩 play

wán 丸 *pill* (*death pulse texture of Large Intestine qi insufficiency*)

wǎn 晚 late

wàn 萬 10,000

wán gǔ 完骨 Mastoid Process, acupoint Gallbladder 12 (Wiseman: Completion Bone)

wán ní 丸泥 *pills of mud* (*death pulse texture of Stomach essence insufficiency*)

wàn wù 萬物 10,000 things, i.e. everything

wáng 亡 perish, collapse, destoryed

wàng 忘 to forget

Wáng Bīng 王冰 (710-805) Tang Dynasty physician whose life work was annotating the Suwen; he spent 12 years on the project

wàng jiàn 妄見 *hallucinate*

wǎng lái 往來 alternating, literally "come and go"

wǎng lái hán rè 往來寒熱 *alternating cold and heat*, from SHL: line 96

wàng mào 妄冒 *frenetic veiling*

wàng xíng 妄行 *frenetic movement*

wàng yán 妄言 *raving*

wàng yán mà lì 妄言罵詈 *rant, rave, curse, scold*

wēi 微 minute, faint, subtle

wéi 為 by, to be/become, as in the capacity of

wéi 維 linking, sustaining/sustainable, maintenance

wéi 危 rooftop (*Chinese constellation*)

wěi 痿 atrophy (Wiseman: wilting)

wěi 疿 unit of measurement for biǎn stone pricking, literally "scar" (Wiseman: bruise or contusion)

wěi 尾 dragontail *(Chinese constellation)*

wèi 謂 is called

wèi 胃 stomach, also a *(Chinese constellation)*

wèi 未 has not yet [happened], also the 8th earthly branch, 1-3pm, 7/7-8/6, year of the Sheep, compass point 210°

wèi 位 position, positions

wěi bì 痿躄 *atrophy lameness* (Wiseman: crippling wilt)

wèi dé qiān zhèng 未得遷正 *(chronobiology term related to running late)*

wèi fēng 胃風 *stomach wind*

wéi gù 為故 for the sake of

wěi hé 委和 compromised harmony *(insufficient wood year name)*

wěi jué 痿厥 *atrophy reversal* (Wiseman: wilting reversal)

wéi mài 維脈 Linking Vessels, 5th and 6th of the 8 Extraordinary Vessels

wèi (qì) 衛(氣) defensive qi, sometimes shortened to defense

wěi yáng 委陽 [Knee] Bend Yang, acupoint Bladder 39

wěi yì 痿易 *atrophy easily*

wèi wǎn 胃脘 stomach [and] digestive cavities, like the extra acupoint at T8 wèiwǎnxiàshū

wèi wǎn yōng 胃脘癰 *stomach/gastric ulcer*

wěi zhēn 微鍼 fine needles, i.e. acupuncture

wěi zhōng 委中 [Knee] Bend Center, acupoint Bladder 40

wēn 溫 warm

wén 聞 hear, smell

wèn 問 ask

wēn bìng 溫病 *warm disease*

wēn nüè 溫瘧 *warm ague* (Wiseman: warm malaria)

wèn yuē 問曰 (v.) asks

wǒ 我 self, I, me, my

wò 握 hold, grip

wò 臥 to lie supine, a euphemism for sleep

wò bù ān 臥不安 *restless sleep*, i.e. waking often

wò bú yù dòng 臥不欲動 lying down with no desire to move, i.e. *listlessness*

wú 無 have not, without, will not

wǔ 五 five

wǔ 忤 insult

wǔ 午 7th earthly branch, 11am-1pm, 6/6-7/6, year of the Horse, noon, summer solstice, compass point 180°, south

wù 霧 fog

wù 物 matter, substance

wù 戊 5th heavenly stem

wù 惡 to be averse to

wù 勿 don't

wù fēng 惡風 *aversion to wind*

wǔ guò 五過 five mistakes

wù hán 惡寒 *aversion to cold*

wū hū 嗚呼 alas

wù jí 物極 things reaching their extreme polarity or end

wù shēng 物生 things generated or born

wù shū wèn 物疎豐 things carelessly crack, i.e. crepitus?

wù táng 鶩溏 *duck slop*, i.e. loose stools?

wǔ wèi 五味 five flavors

wǔ xíng 五行 five elements (Wiseman: five phases)

wǔ yùn 五運 five evolutive phases

wǔ yùn liù qì 五運六氣 five evolutive phases and six climatic factors

wǔ yùn xíng 五運行 five evolutive phase movements

wǔ zàng 五藏 five Zang organs (Unschuld: five depots)

wǔ zhì 五志 five emotions

xī 吸 inhale

xī 膝 knee

xī 息 breathing

xī 西 west

xǐ 喜 joy, happy [event such as a wedding or pregnancy], can also mean tendency for

xì 繫 link

xī bēn 息賁 *breath sprint* (Wiseman: rushing respiration)

xī fēng 西風 west wind

xī jī 息積 *breath accumulation*

xǐ lè 喜樂 joy and music

xī lì 息利 *breathing uninhibited*

xī míng 息鳴 *audible breathing*

xǐ wàng 喜忘 *forgetfulness*

xī yǒu yīn 息有音 breathing has sound, i.e. *breathing audibly*

xià 夏 summer *(season)*

xià 下 below, bottom, lower, inferior, descend, also euphemism for diarrhea or bowel movements

xià gōng 下工 inferior practitioner(s)

xià guān 下關 Lower Gate, acupoint Stomach 7

xià hé xué 下合穴 lower hé-sea point

xià jì 下紀 Lower Record, alternate acupoint name for Ren 4

Xià Jīng 《下經》 Lower Classic

344

xià jù xū 下巨虛 Lower Giant Hollow, acupoint Stomach 39

xià lián 下廉 Lower Ridge, alternate acupoint name of Stomach 39, modern acupoint name of Large Intestine 8

xià shèn 下甚 *extreme precipitation*

xià shū 下俞 lower acupoints, the Nèijīng's name for lower hé-sea points

xià wǎn 下脘 Lower Abdominal Cavity, acupoint Ren 10

xià xiě 下血 *hematochezia* (Wiseman: bloody stool)

xià xiè qīng 下泄清 *diarrhea clear*

xià yǐn shào fù 下引少腹 radiating downward to hypogastrium

xià zhì 夏至 summer solstice *(solar term)*

xiān 先 before, advantage

xián 絃 string of an instrument, i.e. wiry *(pulse texture)*

xián 癇 *seizures* (Wiseman: epilepsy, insanity)

xián 鹹 salty

xián 顯 revelation

xián jīng 癇驚 *seizure shock*

xián jué 癇厥 *seizure reversal*

xián lǚ 弦縷 wire filaments *(death pulse texture of uterus essence insufficiency)*

xiǎn míng 顯明 revealing brightness

xián zhěng 咸整 salty corrections *(transformation of even water year)*

xiāng 相 mutual

xiǎng 響 noise, sound

xiàng 象 image, appearance, elephant

xiàng 項 nape [of the neck]

xiāng chéng 相成 mutual completion

xiāng fù 相傅 minister (Wiseman: assistant)

xiāng shī 相失 mutual loss

xiāo 消 *wasting* (Wiseman: dispersion)

xiǎo 小 small, little, minor

xiào 笑 laugh, smile

xiǎo biàn 小便 urination

xiǎo biàn bì 小便閉 *urinary blockage*

xiào bù xiū 笑不休 *laugh nonstop*

xiǎo chái hú tāng 小柴胡湯 Minor Bupleurum Decoction

xiāo dàn 消癉 *wasting drought* (Wiseman: pure-heat dispersion-thirst)

xiāo huán 消環 *wasting loop*

xiāo kě 消渴 *thirsting and wasting*

xiāo luò 消濼 Disperse Riverbed, acupoint Sanjiao 12

xiāo qì 消氣 *wasting qi*

xiāo shuò 銷鑠 *emaciation*, disperse brilliance *(change of fire)*

xiǎo xīn 小心 small heart <Amy: modern colloquial Chinese for careful>

xiāo zhōng 消中 *wasting center* (Wiseman: center dispersion)

xiě 血 blood

xiè 泄 (n.) [slow dribbly] *diarrhea*, (v.) to leak

xiè 瀉 (n.) [explosive copious] *diarrhea*

xiè 寫 to drain, disperse, reduce <Note from Amy: in modern texts they use the character 瀉 which as far as I can tell means the same thing.>

xié 邪 evil, i.e. pathogen

xiě biàn 血便 *hematochezia*, literally "blood stools"

xiè bù zhǐ 泄不止 *diarrhea nonstop*

xiè fēng 泄風 *diarrhea wind*

xiě jiǎ 血瘕 *blood conglomeration*

xiè yì 解㑊 *lassitude*

xiě kū 血枯 *blood withering* (Wiseman: blood dessication)

xiě nǜ 血衄 *nosebleed*

xiě qì 血氣 blood and qi

xié qì 邪氣 pathogenic qi

xié qì fǎn shèng 邪氣反勝 pathogenic qi overcomes [dominant qi]

xié tòng 脅痛 *rib/hypochondriac pain*

xié xià 脅下 hypochondria, literally "below ribs"

xié xià yǔ yāo bèi xiāng yǐn ér tòng 脅下與腰背相引而痛 *hypochondria radiating to lower/upper back pain*

xiě xiè 血泄 *bloody diarrhea*, i.e. hematochezia

xiě yì 血溢 *blood upwelling*, i.e. epistaxis, hematemesis, hemoptysis

xiè yì 解㑊 *lassitude*

xié zhī mǎn 脅支滿 *rib/armpit fullness* or *rib/propping fullness* <Amy: I'm not sure which>

xiè zhù 泄注 *outpour diarrhea*

xīn 心 heart, also short for dragonheart *(Chinese constellation)*

xīn 新 new

xīn 辛 8th heavenly stem, also spicy *(flavor)*

xìn 顖 fontanel

xīn bì 心痹 *heart impediment*

xīn chè 心掣 *heart pull* (Wiseman: pulling heart)

xìn dǐng fā rè 顖頂發熱 *fontanel expresses heat*

xīn è 辛頞 *burning ethmoid*

xīn fán 心煩 *heart vexation*

xīn fán wǎn 心煩惋 *heart vexation regret*

xīn fēng 心風 *heart wind*

xīn fēng shàn 心風疝 *heart wind hernia*

xīn fù 心腹 heart and abdomen

xīn mǎn 心滿 *heart fullness*

xīn shàn 心疝 *heart hernia* (Wiseman: heart mounting)

xīn tòng 心痛 *heart pain*, i.e. angina

xīn xié tòng 心脇痛 *heart/rib pain*

xīn zào jì 心躁悸 *heart restless/palpitations*

xīng 興 flourish

xíng 刑 punishment, discipline

xíng 形 form (Wiseman: physical body)

xíng 行 walk, travel, move

xíng bì 行痺 *moving impediment*

xǐng kè 省客 questioning guests *(death pulse texture of kidney qi insufficiency)*

xiōng 胸 chest, breast

xióng 雄 male

xiōng fù dà 胸腹大 *chest/abdomen englarged*

xiōng tòng 胸痛 *chest pain*

xiōng xié bào tòng 胸脇暴痛 *chest/ribs violent pain*

xiōng xié zhī mǎn 胸脇支滿 chest [and] ribside propping fullness

xiōng zhōng 胸中 chest center <Amy: I'm not always sure if this means the center of the chest, or the upper and middle jiao.>

xiōng zhōng tòng 胸中痛 *chest center pain*

xiū 休 rest

xiù 秀 fecundate

Xuānyuán 軒轅 a 17 star constellation

xū 虛 empty, deficient (Wiseman: vacuous, vacuity), void

xū 戌 11th earthly branch, 7-9pm, 10/8-11/6, year of the Dog, compass point 300°

xǔ 許 to allow, consent

xū lǐ 虛里 Empty Mile, great connector acupoint of Stomach, located at apical pulse

xū mǎn 虛滿 deficient fullness

xù 序 sequence

xù 蓄 *amassment*

xuān 宣 to announce

xuān 喧 ruckus

xuán 玄 darkness, mystery, void

xuàn mào 眩冒 *dizziness veiling*

xuān míng 宣明 Declare Brightness *(transformation of even metal year)*

xuān píng 宣平 Declare Balance *(transformation of even wood year)*

xuán yōng 懸雍 suspended harmony *(death pulse texture of 12 back-shū insufficiency)*

xué 穴 acupoint, cave, den, hole, cavity, hollow

xùn méng 徇蒙 *sudden dizziness* (Wiseman: clouding giddiness)

xún pū 眴仆 *syncope with dizziness*

yǎ mén 啞門 Mute Door, acupoint Du 15 (Wiseman: Mutes Gate)

yān 焉 particle flagword for an affirmative tone

yān 咽 larynx

yán 言 (n.) words, (v.) to say

yán 炎 inflamed, hot

yǎn 衍 flow to sea

yǎn 演 water flowing long

yàn 晏 late

yǎn dāo 偃刀 upturned blade *(death pulse texture of Cold Heat in the kidney)*

yán shǔ 炎暑 inflamed summerheat, i.e. dog days

yǎn wò 偃臥 sleep/recline supine

yǎng 瘍 sore, ulcer

yáng 陽 sun, i.e. the bright, restless, intangible, energetic, masculine side of Yin and Yang

yáng 揚 flight

yǎng 養 cultivate

yáng 仰 extension, face-up, supine

yáng cì 陽刺 "yang pricking" needling technique: one perpendicular, four surrounding

yáng fǔ 陽輔 Yang Assistant, acupoint Gallbladder 36

yáng jué 陽厥 *yang reversal*

yáng líng quán 陽陵泉 Yang Mound Spring, acupoint Gallbladder 34

yáng shā 陽殺 *yang killing (disease of the 3 spring months)*

Yáng Shàngshàn 楊上善 (585-670) Tang Dynasty author of the Huángdì Nèijīng Tàisù 《黃帝內經太素》 The Yellow Emperor's Internal Classic Grand Basis

yáng wéi 陽維 Yang Linking, 5th of the 8 Extraordinary Vessels

yǎng xī 仰息 *supine audible exhalation*

yáng yōng 陽癰 *yang carbuncle*

yáng zhěn 瘍胗 *lip ulcers*

yángmíng 陽明 yang brightness

yāo 夭 fey, tender (Wiseman: to die young or prematurely)

yào 腰 low back, lumbar

yào 要 key, essential

yào bèi 腰背 lower and upper back

yào dào 要道 essential way (Wiseman: thoroughfare)

yāo gǔ tòng fā 腰股痛發 *low back/buttock pain flares*

yào hài 要害 key vulnerability, vital/crucial point

yāo jǐ shào fù tòng 腰脊少腹痛 *lumbar/hypogastric pain*

yāo jǐ tòng 腰脊痛 *low back/spine pain* (Wiseman: pain in the lumbar spine)

yāo tòng 腰痛 *low back pain* (Wiseman: lumbar pain)

yāo zú qīng 腰足清 *low back/feet cool*

yě 也 particle, usually indicates end of sentence

yè 液 thick [body] fluids

Yè Kěhuá 葉可華 Amy's maternal grandmother

yī 噫 burp, hiccup

yī 衤 garment radical

yí 宜 appropriate, suitable

yí 移 to shift

yí 遺 loss, i.e. involuntary discharge (Wiseman: emission), also (adj.) misplaced or apocryphal, (v.) to lose

yí 頤 cheek/jaw

yí 疑 doubt

yǐ 已 has already [happened]

yǐ 矣 particle for end of sentence, flagword for a completed action

yǐ 以 in order to

yǐ 乙 2nd heavenly stem

yì 亦 also, likewise

yì 嗌 esophagus

yì 異 difference

yì 意 intention, meaning

yì 易 (adj.) easy, (v.) to change

yì 翼 wings *(Chinese constellation)*

yì 抑 constrained

yì bú lè 意不樂 *lack of joy*

yì fǎ 異法 *different methods*

yì gān 嗌乾 *esophageal dryness* (Wiseman: dry throat)

yí nì 遺溺 *enuresis*

yì tòng 嗌痛 *esophageal pain*

yì yǐn 溢飲 *overflow rheum* (Wiseman: spillage rheum)

yì zào 嗌燥 *esophageal dryness*

yì (zhōng) zhǒng 嗌(中)腫 *esophagus swelling*

yīn 陰 shade, i.e. the dark, quiet, tangible, private, feminine, receptive side of Yin and Yang, also euphemism for genitalia

yīn 因 by, because of

yīn 音 sound

yīn 瘖 *aphonia* (Wiseman: loss of voice)

yín 淫 depravity, excess [pathogenic factor]

yǐn 引 to guide/radiate toward, to extend [a muscle or limb]

yǐn 飲 *rheum*, i.e. phlegm-fluid, same character as beverage

yín 寅 3rd earth stem, 3-5am, 2/4-3/5, year of the Tiger, compass point 60°

yǐn bái 隱白 Hermit White, acupoint Spleen 1

yǐn bèi 引背 radiating to upper back

yīn bì 陰痹 *yin impediment*

yín jiāo 齦交 Gum Intersection, acupoint Du 28

yīn jué 陰厥 *yin reversal*

yīn mén 瘖門 Aphonic Door, alternate acupoint name for Du 15

yīn suō 陰縮 *retracted genitals*

yīn yáng 陰陽 the 2 opposing principles in nature and Chinese philosophy

yīn yáng bú cè 陰陽不測 yin and yang cannot be measured

yīn yáng jiāo 陰陽交 *yin-yang exchange* (Wiseman: intermingling of yin and yang)

yīng 膺 also the lateral chest

yíng 營 (adj.) nutritive (Wiseman: construction), (v.) to camp or be encamped

yíng 迎 welcome, greet

yǐng 影 shadow

yìng 應 reflect, echo, resonate, answer to

yīng bèi jiān jiǎ jiān tòng 膺背肩胛間痛 *lateral chest/upper back/scapular pain*

yíng qì 營氣 nutritive qi (Wiseman: construction qi)

yīng shū 膺俞 Lateral-chest Shu, alternate acupoint name for Lung 1

yōng 癰 *carbuncle*

yòng 用 use, function

yōng jū chuāng yáng 癰疽瘡瘍 *carbuncles, abscesses, sores, ulcers*

yǒng quán 湧泉 Bubbling Spring *(death pulse texture of Taiyang qi in muscle insufficiency)*, also acupoint name of Kidney 1

yǒng shuǐ 湧水 *bubbling water*

yōng yáng 癰瘍 *carbuncles and sores*

yōng zhǒng 癰腫 *carbuncle swelling* (Wiseman: welling-abscess)

yóu 猶 as if

yóu 游 to swim

yóu 由 from, to obey/follow, to pass through

yǒu 牖 [latticed] window in a wall that does not have a roof, e.g., window of a walled garden

yǒu 有 to have

yǒu 酉 10th earth branch, 5-7pm, 9/8-10/7, year of the Rooster, compass 270°

yòu 右 right

yóu bù 游部 wandering area

yóu jiān 游間 wanders between

yǒu yú 有餘 extra, literally "to have surplus"

yǒu zǐ 有子 have child, i.e. pregnant

yú 於 preposition: can mean of, from, in, at, to, by, among

yú 余 I

yǔ 與 with, and

yǔ 語 speak, speech, also means *raving* in a pathological context

yǔ 羽 5th note on the musical scale, roughly equivalent to La

yǔ 隅 vertebral height

yù 玉 jade

yù 欲 desire

yù 鬱 *depressed*

yù bǎn 玉版 jade tablet

yú gǔ 髃骨 Clavicle Bone, alternate acupoint name for Large Intestine 15

yù jī 玉機 Jade Mechanism, maybe shorthand for book name Hé Yùjī?

yú jì 魚際 Fish Border, acupoint Lung 10, also the thenar eminence

yù jīng 欲驚 *imminent shock*

yù mào 鬱冒 *depression veiling*

yù shǔ shǔ 玉蜀黍 corn

yù shuǐ 雨水 rain water *(solar term)*

yú yuán shàng wū 踰垣上屋 *climb walls and scale buildings*

yuān 淵 abyss

yuán 源 source

yuán 員 round, circle

yuǎn 遠 distant, distance

yuán qì 元氣 original qi

yuàn wén 願聞 [I am] willing to hear

yuē 曰 says

yuě 噦 belch, burp, belching

yuè 月 moon, month

yuè 樂 music

yuè 躍 jump

yún 雲 cloud(s)

yǔn 隕 to fall from a high place

yùn 運 transport, transportation

yùn (dǒu) 熨(斗) hot iron

yún mén 雲門 Cloud Gate, acupoint Lung 2

yùn yǐn 熨引 hot compresses and guided exercises?

zāi 哉 flagword for exclamations

zài 在 at

zài quán 在泉 At the [Water] Spring, i.e. land qi in six climatic factors terminology which indicates 2nd half of the year, also an alternate acupoint name for Stomach 26

zǎo 早 early

zǎn zhú 攢竹 Savings Bamboo, acupoint Bladder 2 (Wiseman: Bamboo Gathering)

zàng 藏 yin organs (Unschuld: depots, Wiseman: viscera)

zàng fǔ 藏府 internal organs, viscera

zàng xū 藏虛 internal organ deficiency, occurs when erroneously drained during moon waxing

zào 躁 restless, restlessness

zào 燥 dry, dryness

zé 則 (p.) then, (n.) principle

zé lán 澤蘭 bugleweed, lycopi herba (*herb*)

zé xiè 澤瀉 water plantain, alismatis rhizoma (*herb*)

zēng 憎 abhorrence

zēng fēng 憎風 *abhorrence of wind*, extreme wind aversion

zhā 皶 *pimples* (Wiseman: rosacea)

zhàn lì 戰慄 *trembling*

zhān wàng 譫妄 *delirious raving*

zhān yán 譫言 *delirious speech*

zhāng 張 open-net (*Chinese constellation*)

zhǎng 長 (v.) to grow, (n.) elder, eldest

zhāng gōng mì běn 《張公秘本》 Master Zhang's Secret Folio, unpublished version of the Nèijīng by Wáng Bīng's teacher

Zhāng Jièbīn 張介賓 (1563-1642) Ming Dynasty swordsman/doctor, well versed in the Nèijīng and the I Ching, also known as Zhāng Jǐngyuè 張景岳 and Zhāng Shùdì 張熟地 for his use of tonifying herbs, author of the Lèi Jīng 《類經》 Classified Canon (1604)

zhāng xiǎn 彰顯 make conspicuous (*virtue of fire*)

zhào hǎi 照海 Shining Sea, acupoint Kidney 6

zhāo yóu 招尤 *head shaking*

zhàng 服 *distension*

Zhāng Zhòngjǐng 張仲景 (150-219) author of the Shānghán Zábìng Lùn

zhé 蟄 hibernate

zhé 折 to fracture

zhě 者 particle, usually indicates subject or comma

zhé bì 折髀 *fractured femur* (Wiseman: excruciating thigh pain)

zhé chóng 蟄蟲 hibernating insects

zhé yāo 折腰 *fractured lumbar*

zhēn 真 true or truth

zhēn 鍼 needle

zhěn 胗 *pustule*

zhěn 診 diagnosis

zhěn 軫 chariot (*Chinese constellation*)

zhèn 震 thunder *(trigram)*

zhèn 振 to [strive for] rescue

zhèn fā 振發 vibrate release *(change of wood)*

zhěn jīn 疹筋 *papule sinew*

Zhēn Jīng 《鍼經》 Needle Classic, 2nd half of Huangdi Neijing, alternate book name for the Língshū

zhēn rén 真人 true person

zhēn yán 真言 true words

zhēng 蒸 steam

zhēng 徵 4th note on musical scale, roughly equivalent to So; also part of a proof, i.e. sign or symptom

zhēng 爭 conflict(s), at odds with

zhèng 正 upright, proper

zhèng 政 govern, governance

zhèng jì 正紀 proper record(s)

zhèng lì 正立 to stand upright or at attention

zhèng qì 正氣 upright qi (Wiseman: right qi, especially in opposition to disease)

Zhēnjiǔ Jiǎyǐ Jīng 《針灸甲乙經》 ABC's of Acupuncture & Moxibustion by Huángfǔ Mì

zhī 之 subordinate particle that could mean "of ~", indicate possessive, direct object, or end of sentence

zhī 知 know

zhī 支 armpit

zhǐ 止 stop

zhǐ 旨 purpose, aim, imperial decree

zhì 治 to treat, to govern, to prevent from flooding (Wiseman: management)

zhì 痔 *hemorrhoids*

zhì 至 (adj.) ultimate, extreme (v.) to arrive

zhì 志 emotions, willpower, also means [historical] record or document

zhì 痙 *tetany*

zhì 智 wit, wisdom

zhì 制 limit(s)

zhì 滯 *stagnation*

zhì bēi 志悲 emotional grief

zhì běn 治本 treat the root

zhì biāo 治標 treat the branch

zhì bǒ 蹠跛 *sole limp* (Wiseman: metatarsus lameness)

zhì dé 至德 ultimate virtues

zhì jié 治節 governance/organization and moderation/abnegation/conservation/ segmentation (Wiseman: management and regulation)

zhī mǎn 支滿 *armpit/propping fullness*

zhì rén 至人 ultimate person

zhǐ shí 枳實 immature bitter orange (herb)

zhì shù 至數 ultimate numerology

zhī tòng 支痛 *armpit pain*

zhī wěi 肢痿 *limb(s) atrophy*

zhì yì 志意 willpower and intention

zhì yīn 至陰 Ultimate Yin, acupoint Bladder 67, also an alternate name for the longsummer season

zhì zhēn yào 至真要 ultimate truth essentials

zhī zhōu 知周 knowing the big picture

zhōng 中 middle, center

zhōng 終 end

zhōng gǔ 鐘鼓 bells and drums

zhōng gǔ 中古 middle ancient [times]

zhòng hán 中寒 *cold strike*

zhōng jí 中極 Center Pole, acupoint Ren 3 (Wiseman: Central Pole)

zhōng mǎn 中滿 *middle [jiao] fullness*

zhōng qì 中氣 middle [jiao] qi

zhōng qīng 中清 archaic term for gallbladder

zhōng qīng qū xié tòng 中清胠脇痛 *gallbladder/subaxillary/rib pain*

zhōng rè 中熱 *middle [jiao] heat, center heat*

zhōng shū liáo 中俞髎 center acupoint foramen

zhōng wǎn 中脘 Middle Abdominal-Cavity, acupoint Ren 12

zhōng yāng 中央 center, central

zhōng zhèng 中正 justice

zhǒng 腫 swell, swelling

zhòng 眾 crowd, multitude

zhòng fēng 中風 *wind strike*

zhòng gōng 眾工 multitude of practitioners, i.e. everyone

zhǒng shǒu 腫首 *swollen head*

zhòng wù 眾物 multitude of things

zhǒng yāo 腫腰 *swelling in low back*

zhōng yī 中醫 Chinese medicine

zhǒng zhàng 腫脹 *swelling/distension*

zhōu 周 circuit

zhōu dū 州都 wetlands, literally "sandbar capital" (Wiseman: river island official, regional rectifier)

zhōu mì 周密 densely packed

zhòu zhù 驟注 abrupt downpour *(change of earth)*

zhū 諸 all

zhú 朮 atractylodes *(herb)* <Note from Amy: I think this includes both bái zhú and cāng zhú>

zhǔ 主 master/is mastered or governed by, also main, host, or chief [qualities]

zhù 著 (v.) to author, show, prove, (adj.) outstanding

zhǔ qì 主氣 master qi (Wiseman: governing qi, host qi)

zhù xià 注下 *copious watery diarrhea*

zhuǎ 爪 nails, literally "claws"

zhuān 專 focus

zhuǎn 轉 to turn, rotate

zhuǎn yáo 轉搖 turn and sway, i.e. lateral
  rotation/flexion of the spine

zhuì 墜 to fall, plummet

zhuī tòng 膇痛 *lumbar pain*

zhuó 濁 turbid

zhuó 灼 scorch

zhuó bì 着痹 *fixed impediment*

zǐ 子 child, seed, also 1st earthly branch,
  11pm-1am, 12/7-1/5, year of the Rat,
  midnight, winter solstice, compass
  point 0°, north

zì yáng 眥瘍 *sores at canthus*

zōng 宗 ancestor, ancestral [source]

zòng 縱 flaccid lengthwise, literally
  "indulged"

zōng jīn 宗筋 penis, literally "ancestral
  sinew"

zōng qì 宗氣 ancestral qi, i.e. gathering qi

zǒu 走 walk, go

zú 足 foot, leg, sufficient

zú bú rèn shēn 足不任身 *loss of leg function*,
  literally "foot not controlled by body"

zú héng zhǒng 足胻腫 *leg/calf edema*
  (Wiseman: swelling of the foot and
  lower leg)

zú jìng tòng 足脛痛 *leg/shin pain*

zú wěi 足痿 *leg atrophy*

zuǒ 左 left

zuǒ 佐 assist

zuò 作 action

zuò qiáng 做強 strengthener, literally "to
  make/produce strength"

Endnotes

1 天癸 (tiān guǐ): the tenth and last heavenly stem of the (tiān gān) 天干 10 heavenly stems used to designate marks of order and (dì zhī) 地支 12 earthly branches used to denote time (e.g. years, months, days, hours).

2 太沖 (tài chōng): often shortened to Chōng in later books, Tàichōng refers to the Penetrating Vessel, one of the eight extraordinary Vessels. **Acu Trivia!** 太沖 is also the point name of Lv3.

3 任脈 (rèn mài) Controlling Vessel, often mistranslated as "Conception Vessel" 妊脈 (rèn mài).

4 發陳 (fā chén) "release the aged" (i.e. air out stuff that has been sitting around).

5 蕃秀 (fán xiù) "flourish and fecundate."

6 These two lines are followed by (ruò suǒ ài zài wài) 「若所愛在外」, "As if [that which is] beloved is outside." Therefore, I believe "Let all buds come to fruit" and "Let qi be released" are euphemisms for sex. Summer is not just about getting outdoors but also about getting it on.

7 容平 (róng píng) "contain [and] balance," or "tolerate and flatten/suppress."

8 This line is followed by (yǔ jī jù xīng) 「與雞聚興」 "with chickens, gather and flourish," i.e. keep the same sleep schedule as your backyard animals!

9 「使志安寧, 以緩秋刑」 (shǐ zhì ān níng, yǐ huǎn qiū xíng) "Be calm to ease the punishment of autumn."

10 「收斂神氣, 使秋氣平」 (shōu liǎn shén qì, shǐ qiū qì píng) "Withdraw spirit and qi to clear the Lung qi."

11 This is (xiè) 泄 as in slow dribbly diarrhea versus (xiè) 瀉 as in explosive copious diarrhea.

12 閉藏 (bì cáng) "shut and hide," or "closed and hidden."

13 I have been shortening the translation of (shǐ zhì) 使志 "Let the emotions be" to "Be." This line (shǐ zhì ruò fú ruò nì, ruò yǒu sī yì, ruò yǐ yǒu dé) 「使志若伏若匿, 若有私意, 若已有得」 says, "Let the emotions be as if hidden as if concealed, as if harboring secrets, as if [you have] already made gains."

14 Do not open the (pí máo) 皮毛 "skin and pores" which causes the qi to be (jí duó) 亟奪 ...urgently taken? Robbed? It is the same (duó) 奪 as "give and do not take" in spring taboos.

15 ...like a mummy?

16 俞 (shū): according to the second oldest dictionary of Chinese characters, the *Shuō Wén Jiě Zì* (SWJZ) 俞 is a character for "a boat of hollowed wood" (i.e. a canoe?) Here it means any general acupoint. Because it looks like the last name Yú 俞, this character is often mispronounced by non-practitioners.

17 "Back" refers specifically to (bèi) 背 "upper back," not (yāo) 腰 "low back" or (jǐ) 脊 "spine."

18 中央 (zhōng yāng) "center"... just center. No wind is attached to it, versus the 4 Winds that precede it, (dōng fēng) 東風, (nán fēng) 南風, (xī fēng) 西風, (běi fēng) 北風.

19 Short for "...and also stores jīng-essence in ~" (this line occurs after orifices but is the same Zang).

20 二陰 (èr yīn): the urethral orifice and anus.

21 黍 (shǔ): some translations say "glutinous millet"; this is also a character that shows up in (shǔ shǔ) 蜀黍 "sorghum" and (yù shǔ shǔ) 玉蜀黍 "corn," i.e. "jade sorghum," introduced to Asia in the 14th Century.

22 Short for "Therefore [the practitioner] knows disease occurs at ~."

23 Includes both (pí) 皮 "skin," the same character as (chén pí) 陳皮 "aged tangerine skin," and (máo) 毛 "fur," which means body hair

and pores—all the other body parts are only a single character: (jīn) 筋 "sinew," (mài) 脈 "vessel," (ròu) 肉 "flesh," (gǔ) 骨 "bone."

24 Though not entirely historically accurate, I have chosen the notes closest to the seven-note diatonic scale a contemporary practitioner might recognize: (gōng) 宮 "Do," (shāng) 商 "Re," (jiǎo) 角 "Mi," (zhēng) 徵 "So," (yǔ) 羽 "La." The ancient Chinese scale was a five-note pentatonic scale not specific to any key.

25 Here is the passage that connects Liver with emotional health! (Huà) 化 "transformation" generates (wǔ wèi) 五味 the "five flavors." (Dào) 道 "The Way" generates (zhì) 智 "wit" or "wisdom." (Xuán) 玄 The mystical "darkness" generates (shén) 神 the ineffable "spirit," which in weather is wind, on land is wood, and so on.

26 I.e. the land of Tàichōng. The sage stands facing south. In front is (guǎng míng) 廣明 "broad brightness," behind is (tài chōng) 太沖. **Acu Trivia!** This is the same Great Rushing as the acupoint name of Lv3., 太沖.

27 Ends at (mìng mén) 命門 "Life Gate," an alternate name for (jīng míng) 睛明 "Eyeball Brightness," UB1. **Acu Trivia!** Today, (mìng mén) 命門 is the name of Du4.

28 Taiyin is below Guangming, which goes up from the center of the torso.

29 Center of yin whose Chong is below.

30 Homonym alert! This is a different character (jué) 絕 from that of (jué yīn) 厥陰. 絕 (jué): "ending" or "termination" versus 厥 (jué): *Reversal.*

31 死不治 (sǐ bú zhì) "death, not treatable," i.e. fatal.

32 *Carbuncle Swelling* occurs below.

33 辟陰 (pì yīn): literally *Split yin.* Fatal.

34 節 (jié): solar terms, regularity, seasonal nodes, joints, holidays, moderation, governance, and regulation... I am guessing that the Lung is in charge of interfacing between the body and the 24 Solar Terms, since it interacts most directly with seasonal weather changes. Giovanni Maciocia's book The Foundations of Chinese Medicine (volume 3, p.132) goes with regulation, although, if we want the format

to match, perhaps (zhì jié) 治節 means "governance/organization and moderation/abnegation," as that fits with metal.

35 膻中 (dàn zhōng) "Chest Center." **Acu Trivia!** Also the name of R17. Often mispronounced as shān zhōng. Shān is how you pronounce the character 膻 when it means the smell of mutton or goat.

36 日 (rì): the character for "sun" which indicates day, the way that (yuè) 月 "moon" indicates month.

37 候 (hòu): the character for "wait" which originally meant "to observe the changes of atmospheric conditions," or "to hold in readiness," as in what servants do for their masters, or what a good host does for guests. Here it means a five-day week.

38 Includes (zhé) 蟄 "hibernate," (fēng) 封 "seal," and (cáng) 藏 "hide."

39 Filled at sinews to generate blood and qi, of sour flavor, of blue-green color.

40 Qi Bo does not actually say "Fu" here, but lists: Spleen, Stomach, Large Intestine, Small Intestine, San Jiao, Bladder.

41 Lips and (sì bái) 四白 "Four White," the ancient anatomical term for sclera. **Acu Trivia!** (Sì bái) 四白 is the name of St2.

42 Ultimate Yin, not within anything.

43 關格 (guān gé) "Block and Repel": (guān) 關 "urinary stoppage" and (gé) 格 "continuous vomiting". It seems like (gé) 隔 from Chapter 7 and (gé) 格 here both mean continuous vomiting.

44 If Juyang extreme then [disease] enters Kidney.

45 If Jueyin extreme then [disease] enters Liver.

46 Red pulse arrives also panting? (is this a symptom or a pulse texture?) and hard 「赤脈之至也喘而堅。」 (chì mài zhī zhì yě chuǎn ér jiān).

47 White pulse arrives panting and floating, empty above and solid below. 「白脈之至也喘而浮, 上虛下實。」 (bái mài zhī zhì yě chuǎn ér fú, shàng xū xià shí).

48 肺痹寒熱 (fèi bì hán rè) *Lung Impediment Cold Heat* ... I am not sure if this is one combined disease name, or two disease names.

49 Blue-green pulse arrives long and bounces from left to right.

50 Yellow pulse arrives large and empty.

51 厥疝 (jué shàn) *Reversal Hernia*. Not an *Impediment*.

52 Black pulse arrives top, hard and large.

53 Lone pulse is counterflow. Deficient is following.

54 According to the annotations in Unschuld p.259, (săn shū) 散俞 "scattered points" are āshì points scattered along the meridian that are not any of the (běn shū) 本輸 "original transporters," i.e. the five shū-points (jǐng-well, yíng-spring, shū-stream, jīng-river, hé-sea). Wang Bing calls them "holes far apart."

55 Unschuld p.259: "parting structures between muscles and flesh... [layers] where, if pierced, blood appears."

56 Unschuld p.260: "transporters on the network [vessels]."

57 淫 (yín) "depravity" or "excess," the character for the six pathogenic factors, same as in Chapter 9's 氣淫 (qì yín) "qi excess" where overacting occurs before its proper time/season.

58 「蟄蟲周密，君子居室。」 (zhé chóng zhōu mì, jūn zǐ jū shì). "[When] hibernating insects [are] densely packed, the superior man stays indoors." I have a mental image of a wise goatee'd Confucian gentleman making himself cozy with a book and a lamp, perfectly aligned with the season just like the insects, while the foolish engage in snowsports and other outdoor activities. The other hibernating insect lines do not have such tips.

59 Unschuld and many other scholars believe this is copying error that should read (xiāo kě) 消渴 *Wasting and Thirsting*, i.e. diabetes. I agree.

60 Liver pulse hard and long, complexion not green.

61 溢飲 (yì yǐn) *Overflow Rheum*: [disease of] violent thirst, copious drinking, easily enters muscle and skin outside the gut and stomach.

62 Stomach pulse hard and long, complexion red.

63 Spleen pulse hard and long, complexion yellow.

64 「腰脊痛而身有痹也。」 (yāo jǐ tòng ér shēn yǒo bì yě): "Low back/spine pain and body has (bì) 痹 *Impediment*."

65 Diseases of corresponding Zang: spring/Liver, summer/Heart, longsummer/Spleen, autumn/Lung, winter/Kidney.

66 Therefore, blood drains and qi moves easily.

67 精 (jīng): I did not know this character could be used as a verb. I think it probably means "to distill into" here.

68 Double Excess = blood and qi overflow + blood stasis in Luò-collaterals.

69 Since no point names are specified, there is disagreement on which specific points this passage refers to. Zhāng Jièbīn 張介賓 believes these to be UB42–46, while Mǎ Shì 馬蒔 and many other commentators believe they are Du9–12 (with an unnamed Du point beneath the fourth vertebra).

70 志 (zhì): This is the same character as the (wǔ zhì) 五志 "five emotions", and willpower, the emotion attributed to Kidney.

71 This is the same character (pò) 迫 from Chapter 9, a deficiency that does not arrive at the expected time.

72 Kidney qi abundant + work in water = Taiyang qi weakens [therefore] Kidney fat withers and cannot fill bones with marrow, [which leads to] one water (Kidney) being unable to defeat two fires (Liver + Heart); thus cold goes into bones.

73 Neither sensation nor function = body and willpower disconnected. This is called death.

74 Nutritive qi 榮氣 (róng qì) deficient = 不仁 (bù rén) "no sensation." Defensive qi 衛氣 (wèi qì) deficient = 不用 (bú yòng) "no function."

75 Qi Bo quotes from the (xià jīng) 下經 <u>Lower Classic</u>: 「胃不和則臥不安。」 (wèi bù hé zé wò bù ān) "Stomach disharmony creates unpeaceful sleep."

76 Bloodletting technique on UB40.

77 The text here just says "Foot Shaoyang" without specifying a location on the channel.

78 In extreme cases [patient] will retch easily.

79 Similarly, the text here says to needle Foot Jueyin without specifying a point.

80 I think this means (bā xié) 八邪 "eight evils," the extra points in the finger webbing.

81 There is a special note here that says the two sublingual veins = (lián quán) 廉泉, R23.

82 風瘧 (fēng nuè) *Wind Ague.*

83 肺消 (fèi xiāo) *Lung Wasting*: drink one urinate two, death, no treatment.

84 湧水 (yǒng shuǐ) *Bubbling Water*: abdomen not hard on palpation, (shuǐ qì) 水氣 "water qi" in LI, sloshes when walking briskly like leather bag of sauce. A disease of water.

85 死不可治 (sǐ bù kě zhì) "fatal, cannot be treated."

86 口麋 (kǒu mí) *Oral Putrefaction*: Diaphragm and Intestine separation leads to constipation, rises up to become this condition.

87 食亦 (shí yì) *Food Changes*: eat more but lose weight.

88 鼻淵 (bí yuān): turbid *Nasal Discharge* without cease, can become *Fatal Nosebleed* 衄衊瞑目 (nǜ miè míng mù).

89 If laterally rotate, then hypochondriac fullness occurs.

90 Sanjiao cough "gathers in Stomach, relates to Lung, causing [the patient] to have copious nasal discharge, spittle, facial edema and qi counterflow."

91 「得炅則痛立止」 (dé jiǒng zé tòng lì zhǐ) "Apply warmth and pain will cease instantly."

92 (hán qì) 寒氣 "Cold qi" and (jiǒng) 炅 "warmth/firelight" battle, filling vessels.

93 Applying pressure dispels the stagnant blood and qi, relieving the pain.

94 沖脈 (chōng mài) Penetrating Vessel which "begins at R4, ascends vertically along the abdomen."

95 Apply pressure and (rè) 熱 "heat" qi arrives, relieving the pain.

96 When qi returns, then [patient] revives.

97 In extreme cases, this can cause (ǒu xiě) 嘔血 *Hematemesis* and (sūn xiè) 飧泄 *Lienteric Diarrhea*.

98 Huángfǔ Mì thinks that minerals create (jū) 疽 *Abscess* and that (chēn) 瘨 is a copying error. In all the other instances *Withdrawal* is mentioned as (diān) 癲. I agree with him.

99 痏 (wěi): literally "scar." I think this is a unit of measurement for biǎn stone pricking.

100 腠理 (còu lǐ): technically, this is the interstices.

101 Also known as (zàng fǔ zhī fēng) 藏府之風 *Wind of Zang/Fu*.

102 Most interesting. I never thought of (wěi) 痿 *Atrophy* as being caused by *Heat*.

103 On *Vessel Atrophy*: 「脈痿, 樞折挈, 脛縱而不任地也」 (mài wěi, shū zhé qiè, jìng zòng ér bú rèn dì yě). "Pivots fractured by convulsion, shins flaccid and unable to touch the ground."

104 According to Qi Bo, "In spring and summer there is more yang qi and less yin qi. In autumn and winter there is abundant yin qi and frail yang qi." 「春夏則陽氣多而陰氣少, 秋冬則陰氣盛而陽氣衰。」 (chūn xià zé yáng qì duō ér yīn qì shǎo, qiū dōng zé yīn qì shèng ér yáng qì shuāi).

105 This is (jué nì) 厥逆 Reversal Counterflow versus (jué) 厥 Reversal in the last table.

106 It actually says (shǒu xīn zhǔ) 手心主 "Hand Heart Master" here, which equals what we call Hand Jueyin Pericardium today.

107 10 (fēn) 分 equals 1 (qián) 錢, approximately 3.75 grams.

108 The text does not specify (bái zhú) 白朮 or (cāng zhú) 蒼朮.

109 This is the same character 蘭 as in (zé lán) 澤蘭 or (pèi lán) 佩蘭.

110 This is the same character (chén) 陳 "aged" as in (chén pí) 陳皮.

111 If pulse does not arrive, presents as (yīn) 瘖 *Aphonia*, no treatment is necessary.

112 Patient "will not know to speak with people" 「不知與人言」 (bù zhī yǔ rén yán).

113 Questioning guests (xng kè) 省客 pulse: congested and drum.

114 If Shaoyin [pulse] does not arrive, *Reversal*.

115 Wáng Bīng 王冰 and Lǐ Guóqīng 李國清 agree that (yuè) 躍 means "to jump" but commentators disagree on whether this is a clerical error with no meaning or a condition name that has been lost.

116 *Tendency to Anger* (shàn nù) 善怒 is known as *Tortured Reversal* (jiān jué) 煎厥.

117 「血見於鼻」 (xiě jiàn yú bí). Ctext.org has the character (xiě) 血 "blood" here so it could also mean hemoptysis coming out of the nostrils, but I think the line refers to (nǜ) 衂 *Nosebleed*.

118 Although Unschuld translates (zhèn) 振 as "blossoming," (zhèn) 振 is actually a verb that means "to rescue," or "to strive for rescue." It has connotations of arousal and is a homonym for (zhèn) 震, the trigram for "thunder," which strikes the earth to arouse all the hibernating insects, beginning the process of life generation that includes blossoming.

119 "In the 72 days at the end of four seasons" (i.e. 18 days' transition belonging to earth after Solar Terms(lì chūn) 立春 "start of spring," (lì xià) 立夏 "start of summer," (lì qiū) 立秋 "start of autumn," (lì dōng) 立冬 "start of winter").

120 腦戶 (nǎo hù) "Brain Window."

121 仆 (pū) "fall [forward]," i.e. faint.

122 脫色 (tuō sè) "desertion of complexion," i.e. blanch.

123 氣街 (qì jiē) "Qi Street."

124 傴 (qū) "humpback."

125 根蝕 (gēn shí) *Root Corrosion*.

126 缺盆 (quē pén) "Chipped Basin." **Acu Trivia!** St12, also the anatomical term for the supraclavicular fossa.

127 魚際 (yú jì) "Fish Border." **Acu Trivia!** Lu10, the anatomical term for the thenar eminence.

128 客主人 (kè zhǔ rén) "guest/master."

129 See Chapter 9.

130 Do not hit bone when needling *Sinew Impediment*.

131 Do not hit sinew or bone when needling *Muscle Impediment*. If [the practitioner] harms the sinew and bone, ulcers will develop.

132 癲病 (diān bìng) *Epilepsy*: disease occurs once a year at onset, then once a month if untreated, then 4–5 times a month if untreated.

133 窗 (chuāng) = window in a dwelling. 牖 (yǒu) = window in a wall (SWJZ).

134 膺 (yīng) = lateral chest area. 胸 (xiōng) = central chest area (SWJZ).

135 Prefrontal 5 = Du24, GB13, St8. I did not know the *Nèijīng* included scalp acupuncture! This is not the Jiāo 焦 style reflexology scalp acupuncture I learned in school.

136 䲰骨 (qiú gǔ): literally "nasal congestion bone." I think this is the zygoma.

137 沖疝 (chōng shàn) *Rushing Hernia* is a "disease which starts at the lower jiao and rushes up toward the Heart, [creating] pain with constipation/urine retention."

138 Wáng Bīng 王冰 thinks the central bony foramen of the Yangming is St36; Zhāng Jièbīn 張介賓 thinks it is the shū-stream point St43; and Yáng Shàngshàn 楊上善 believes it is St37 (i.e. the middle of the three lower hé-sea points St36, St37, and St39, which are all shū-transporters on the Yangming channel).

139 Retain needles for long time if (hán) 寒 "cold" is present.

140 This chapter begins without preamble, but here the Emperor states, "[I am] willing to hear explanations."

141 蓋 (gài) "to cover," as with a lid.

142 藏 (cáng) "to hide," as with treasure, the same character as Zang.

143, 144, 145   My computer refuses to type the (lǚ) (月呂) that means "paraspinal muscles" as one character, so I have opted for (lǚ) 膂 which also has the flesh radical and means "backbone" here.

146 These are constellations from the 28 Mansions of Chinese astronomy.

147 眚 (shěng) "calamity," originally a character for a growth 生 on the eye 目 (SWJZ).

148 隕 (yǔn) "to fall from a high place," like a shooting star.

149 Actually, it is 60 days and 87.5 (kè) 刻 Quarter Hours, so 60 days and 21.87 hours, almost but not quite 61 days.

150 「化氣不政, 生氣獨治，雲物飛動, 草木不寧」 (huà qì bù zhèng, shēng qì dú zhì, yún wù fēi dòng, cǎo mù bù níng) "If there is not enough Transformation to balance Generation there will be too much flying movement in the clouds and no serenity in the woods" and *Rib Pain with Severe Vomiting* occurs instead.

151 血溢 (xiě yì) "bleeding from the upper orifices," i.e. epistaxis, hematemesis, hemoptysis.

152 「藏氣伏, 化氣獨治」 (cáng qì fú, huà qì dú zhì) "Hiding qi [is] hidden, transforming qi governs alone." No storage, only transformation.

153 If (sù) 肅 "silence" and (shā) 殺 "killing" are extreme, then *Body Heaviness, Vexation Grievance, Chest Pain Radiating to Upper Back*, and *Bilateral Rib Fullness with Pain Radiating to Hypogastrium* occur, reflecting Venus.

154 If withdrawal is severe and Generation descends/declines, then *Panting, Cough, Counterflow Qi, Shoulder/Upper Back Pain*, and *Sacrum/ Genital/Buttock/Knee/Hip/Calf/Shin/Leg Disease* occur.

155 In extreme cases.

156 「民乃康」 (mín nǎi kāng) "People recover from diseases."

157 「收氣乃後」 (shōu qì nǎi hòu) "Withdrawal qi is delayed."

158 四維 (sì wéi): either "all directions" or the 4 ordinal directions (NE, NW, SE, SW). This is the same (wéi) 維 character as the (wéi mài) 維脈 Linking Vessels.

159 平氣 (píng qì) "even qi."

160 不及 (bù jí) "insufficient," i.e. not reaching.

161 太過 (tài guò) "excess," i.e. too [far] past.

162 端 (duān) "standing upright" (SWJZ).

163 衍 (yǎn): originally meaning "flow to sea" (SWJZ), this is the sort of flooding that enriches the soil of a delta or other flat piece of land, like the seasonal silt deposits of the Nile.

164 流 (liú) "water moving" (SWJZ).

165 演 (yǎn) "water flowing long" (SWJZ).

166 炎 (yán) "hot," same character as inflammation, with 2 fires stacked on top of each other.

167 溽 (rù) "damp summerheat" (SWJZ).

168 令 (lìng) "to express commands" (SWJZ).

169 清 (qīng): this is the character for "clear" but I have concluded that in the *Sùwèn* it often means "cool."

170 實 (shí): this is the same character as "excess" or "solid" but here it means "fruit part" like (guā lóu shí) 瓜蔞實.

171 裡急 (lǐ jí) *Tenesmus*.

172 支滿 (zhī mǎn) *Propping Fullness*.

173 瞤 (rún) *Eye Twitch*.

174 瘈 (chì) *Clonic Convulsion*.

175 否 (pǐ): hexagram 8 from the *I Ching*, homonym to the later character (pǐ) 痞 for glomus.

176 欬 (kài) "sound of counterflow qi" (SWJZ), old character for (ké) 咳 "cough."

177 厥 (jué) *Reversal*.

178 Here we see the shamanic roots of Chinese medicine, in the different colored (shī guǐ) 屍鬼 "corpse ghosts" that (fàn) 犯 "offend," "attack," or "invade" deficiencies.

179 I have added the word "year" here to be faithful to the text, although it is omitted in the other entries in the table.

180 膻中 (dàn zhōng) "chest center." **Acu Trivia!** This is also the name of R17, often mispronounced as shān zhōng.

181 「不司氣化」 (bù sī qì huà) "[does] not transform [based on] dominant qi."

182 Instead of between qi, Shaoyin has (jū qì) 居氣 "resident qi."

183 If extreme Damp ascends to create Heat, treat with bitter warm, envoy with sweet spicy, and stop when sweating is achieved.

184 冷 (lěng).

185 「以和為利」 (yǐ hé wéi lì) "Harmonize to benefit."

186, 187 冷 (lěng).

188 For *Shaoyin Retaliation*, astringe with sour, release with spicy bitter, and soften with salty.

189 For *Shaoyang Retaliation*, use warm/hot herbs, with similar method as *Shaoyin Retaliation*.

190 維 (wéi): Extraordinary Vessels Yin Wei and Yang Wei.

Index

Wiseman, N., 139, 144
withdrawal/mania, 127
Wood, 247
    insufficient years, 272

yang qi, 26
    pathogenic factors that
        deplete, 27
    sun cycle and, 28
Yang Reversal, 173
Yangming, 42
    blood/qi preponderance, 108
    commonalities of disease, 279
    death presentations, 80
    directional energetics, 245
    diseases and pulse pictures, 183–4
    seasonal disease etiology, 230
Yangming reversal, 171
Yangming Vessel, 126

Yellow Emperor, 20
yin yang
    definitions and functions, 34–6
    differentiating, 304
    disease location/season and, 32
    hand and foot channels, 109
    imbalances, 38
    in pulse reading, 43
    of sky qi, 241
    Spleen and Stomach, 123
    sun cycle and, 32
yin yang reflection images, 34
ying pulse, 93

Zang and Fu organs, 59
Zhang Zhongjing, 128